BEHIND CLOSED DOORS:

a journey through manic depression

by

Carol Davis

In love with Christ
Carol Davis

Xulon PRESS

Printed in the United States of America

ISBN 9781624195518

Acknowledgement

*T*hank you to Crystal, Kristi, Amy and Lorraine that met with me during the Crown Financial Seminar meetings three years ago. Your encouragement has birthed this book. Thank you to Cindy who told me I could write about anything if I had the right motive. Thank you to the ladies who had special prayer for me in the prayer room; your accountability has kept me on track. Thank you to Sandra for sharing her testimony with me to put in the book. Thank you does not seem enough for Bro. Randy and Pam who have been such an encouragement to me; I love and appreciate them greatly. Thank you to all the doctors, psychiatrists, and counselors I had over the years that have brought me out of deep depressions and back down from manic. Thank you to Dr. Snowden who not only listens but talks to me. Thank you to Carolyn, my prayer partner, my sister in Christ, you do much in my life, much. You think you cannot do much for the Kingdom of Christ, but you encourage me a lot. Our prayer times are special to me as I know they are to you. You have brought laughter and joy into my life. You are a bright spot in my day. Let your light shine as Jesus shines through you. Thank you to Momma who stood up to the doctors and nurses and told them I was not faking. She taught me names to faces and events after I had electric shock treatments. Thank you to Daddy who listened; he did not know what to say, but he was there. Thank you to Nanny and Pa, they taught me unconditional love. Nanny's one of my best friends, and I cherish our times together. We talk about the LORD, and Jesus is my favorite subject. We may not always agree with each other, but that is okay, too. Thank you to Johnnie and Kathleen our church secretaries you have been a big help in advice for the book and printing it so I could proof it. Thank you to Nancy, Al, Tracie, Norma and Jim for listening and talking to me, they are great friends, and they help me on Wednesdays when I cook for the Fellowship Suppers. Thank you to my church family for your prayers, support and love for me. Thank you to all who helped cook last year when I could not. Thank you to all those who serve the food and clean up the kitchen and fellowship hall afterwards, I could not do Fellowship Suppers without you. Thank you to my daughter and son, Jen and Jay and their families; they keep me young and are priceless treasures in my life. My life would be so empty without them. Thank you to the other people in other churches who have prayed for me. Thank You to my sisters-in-law, Cindy and Dee Dee, my brothers, Dewayne and Bryan, all my family and all Buh's family — you make my life full.

I want to give a special thank you to Meda Carol for designing the cover for the book.

Thank you to you who read this book. You have been a part of the healing process. Thank you to Pat and Pat who are always there to listen and talk.

Thank You, God, that You are real and true and alive. Every word of the Bible can be counted on. The Bible is tested and tried and proved by so many who have come before me, and will prove so to those who come after me. Thank You, God, for Your love, Your mercy and Your grace, thank You for Your forgiveness. In Jesus Name, Amen.

(1)

God is a Good Shepherd

ॐ

*T*he following are some questions I wrote when I first started writing this book. I do not have all the answers, but God does. Seek Him while he can be found. You have today with no promise of tomorrow. Part of the following is what Jimmy, our youth minister, wanted to share at the Christmas Eve service at church. It was snowed out, so we did not have the service, but he gave me permission to use it here in the book. Some of you are hurting right now. Holidays are especially tough for the depressed and broken hearted. Maybe you are hurting due to a separation or even a divorce of your spouse.Maybe there are various problems in your family; troubles with friends or other loved ones. Maybe you are even dealing with failing health. Maybe it is the loss of a job or the uncertainty of your future. Whatever your situation, *God knows, God cares and God understands*. Most of all, He loves you still. He offers us the encouragement we need through His Word. We find comfort in the 23rd Psalm in the promises of the Bible. The words are God's provision to believers in Christ.

Verse 1 *The LORD is my shepherd;* — if the LORD is my shepherd

Is the LORD your shepherd? Are you trying to navigate life all on your own? Try looking at God's road map called the Bible.

Verse 1 *I shall not want.* — not have unmet needs

Does God give us everything that we need? God gives us even some of our wants. God can create in us desires only He can fill.

Verse 2 *He makes me to lie down in green pastures;* — rest and provision

Does God invite us to have times of rest? We do not have to sleep to rest. What happens when you get still before God?

Verse 2 *He leads me beside still waters.* — directs my going to peaceful places

Jesus can still calm the storms in our lives. Does He always make the storm go away? Have you stopped and told Him there is a storm? God can calm His child in the storm or He can calm the storm.

Verse 3 *He restores my soul;* — refreshment

Will you let Him? Obey what He asks you to do. God listens to every word we say or think. God knows our heart and really understands.

Verse 3 *He leads me in paths of righteousness For His name's sake.*

Does that path sometimes lead us through times of depression? God can lead us then out of that depression. Does He do it just so He can get the glory from it? Give God the credit when He heals you.

Verse 4 *Yea, though I walk through the valley of the shadow of death,* — low places

Can a shadow hurt you? Is it all right to go down into a valley? Death does not always refer to dying; it can also apply to depression. God can remove clouds of depression. He does it on His time table.

Verse 4 *I will fear no evil;* — not be afraid

Are you responsible for your depression? Is it your fault you are depressed? God is in control,

Verse 4 *For You are with me;* — never alone

God is with you all the time. God is with you even when you cannot see Him. God is with you even when you cannot feel Him.

Verse 4 *Your rod and Your staff, they shall comfort me* — encouragement

Is it all right for God to correct you? Will you let God discipline you in love? Ask God hard questions, expecting His still small voice to answer. Look for His Words of leadership in the Bible.

Verse 5 *You prepare a table before me in the presence of my enemies;* —provision

Will you invite Jesus to sit with you next time you sit down to eat a meal? Take time to pray and spend a few moments talking to God before you eat. Are you afraid of the enemy?

Verse 5 *You anoint my head with oil;* — oil represents healing and the Holy Spirit

Will you ask to be filled with the Holy Spirit? Do not be afraid of the Holy Spirit. The Holy Spirit is your Helper.

Verse 5 *My cup runs over.* — abundance of supplies
>   Do you have as much of God as you want? You can have as much of God as you need. Allow the Holy Spirit to spill out of you onto the people God places in your life.

Verse 6 *Surely goodness and mercy shall follow me* — as God leads
>   Do you want the Good Shepherd to follow you anywhere you go? God is good all the time. Allow Him to show you His mercy, His grace, His goodness, His forgiveness and His love.

Verse 6 *All the days of my life* — promised hope
>   Will you promise two people today that you will allow God to be the one who decides when your life is to end? Think about how many days you have left on this earth. Decide right now that you want Jesus in all your days.

Verse 6 *And I will dwell in the house of the LORD*
>   Can you say it has been good when you walk out the door of your church? You make it a better place. Will you find a place in your home where you and God can be alone together, where He can meet with you on a daily basis?

Verse 6 *Forever* — promised inheritance
>   Eternity lives in your heart. You were made for something besides what you see here on earth. If you cannot comprehend all this now, would you ask someone, even God Himself to help you understand? Today—if you are depressed enough to think of taking your own life, tell someone who cares, someone who can help you get better.

(2)

God Calls it Lying

🌰

*O*ver the years I stretched the truth. God calls it lying. So now I call it lying. I lied because I thought it made a story sound better. But God has taught me I have to tell the truth in love. When in doubt now, I tell the truth. The truth makes a stronger story. Lying hurt me. It was a sin against God and separated me from God; all sin separates us from God. It hurts others. They did not know what to believe of what I said.

Blessed be the LORD my Rock, who trains my hands for war, And my fingers for battle—Psalm 144:1 (NKJV)

Good and bad people are going to go to hell if you and I do not tell them about Jesus. They are not going to come to our churches. We have to go to them, into their homes or work-place and into their lives.

The people answered Him, "We have heard from the law that the Christ remains forever; and how can You say, 'The Son of Man must be lifted up'? Who is this Son of Man?" Then Jesus said to them, "A little while longer the light is with you. Walk while you have the light, lest darkness overtake you; he who walks in darkness does not know where he is going. While you have the light, believe in the light, that you may become sons of light." These things Jesus spoke, and departed, and was hidden from them. But although He had done so many signs before them, they did not believe Him, that the word of Isaiah the prophet might be fulfilled, which he spoke: "Lord, who has believed our report? And to whom has the arm of the LORD been revealed?" Therefore they could not believe, because Isaiah said again: "He has blinded their eyes and hardened their hearts, Lest they would see with their eyes, Lest they should understand with their hearts and turn, So that I should heal them." These things Isaiah said when he saw His glory and spoke of Him. Nevertheless even among the rulers many believed in Him, but because of the Pharisees they did not confess Him, lest they should be put out of the synagogue; for they loved the praise of men more than the praise of God. Then Jesus cried out and said, "He who believes in Me, believes not in Me but in Him who sent Me. And he who sees Me sees Him who sent Me. I have come as a light into the world that whoever believes in Me should not abide in darkness. And if anyone hears My words and does not believe, I do not judge him; for I did not come to judge the world but to save the world. He who rejects Me, and does not receive My words, has that which judges him—the word that I have spoken will judge him in the last day. For I have not spoken on my own authority; but the Father who sent Me gave Me a command, what I should say and what I should speak. And I know that His command is everlasting life. Therefore, whatever I speak, just as the Father has told Me, so I speak." John 12:34-50 (NKJV)

Abba, forgive me for lying in my past. Over the years You have taught me truth is stranger than fiction. I do not have to embellish anything that has happened or happens to me. But, I need to tell the truth in love. Abba, forgive me for all the times when I knew it was 5, and I would say it was 6 because I thought it made a better story. Your truth, God's Word, and me telling Your truth is imperative. I have to tell the truth, the whole truth and nothing but the truth, so help me God.

Abba, You say soldiers of Christ fight best on their knees. Teach my fingers to fight and my hands to war. In Jesus Name, Amen.

(3)

"Write"

🙶

I did not know what to write when God started urging me to write. I did not know what to write about. God told me to "**write**." I started with a few paragraphs; it still did not come together. But then God said, "**Write to Stephen Curtis Chapman**," and the words just flowed. Billie proof read it, and now I am making corrections. I do not know what to do with my story. I just know I am to send my testimony to Stephen Curtis Chapman. I praise and thank my God for what He has done in my past and continues to do in my life; I praise Him for the good and the bad. I praise God now in the midst of this manic depression. I praise and thank Him that I am even alive. I started writing the book Tuesday night, August 12, 2008. I wrote my testimony and sent it to Stephen Curtis Chapman. That was the beginning of this book. I went back into my journals to find the dated materials I have included in the book. I wrote from my heart; I hope to your heart.

Restlessness birthed this book. Restlessness led me many years ago to go to the three year old Sunday school room to volunteer to teach. I have been teaching them ever since. I am not sure all restlessness is sin. Restlessness also kept me on the go. I was always making trips to town, never satisfied just to be in one place. Always I wanted to be somewhere else, doing something else. I was never satisfied to be where I was at the moment. I used a lot of gas just going, never satisfied with where I was or what I was doing. I think peace; God's peace is the answer to my sin of restlessness. I need to be content with what God gives me each day. He is more than enough for me.

Be anxious for nothing, but in everything by prayer and supplication, with thanksgiving, let your requests be made known to God; and the peace of God, which sur- passes all understanding, will guard your hearts and minds through Christ Jesus. Philippians 4:6-7 (NKJV)

Let the words of my mouth and the meditations of my heart Be acceptable in Your sight, O LORD, my strength and my Redeemer. Psalm 19:14 (NKJV)

Abba, forgive me for being restless. Help me rest securely in Your love and protection, knowing nothing comes to me except it comes through You. Thank You for restlessness. Thank You for peace. You used both at different times in my life. Both brought me into a closer relationship with You. I praise You. Thank You for a peace that passes all under- standing and that peace comes only from You, God. Help me enjoy just being with You wherever You put me, whatever You want me to do. Help me plan wisely when I go to town to get everything done in one trip. Help me remember what I am sup- posed to be doing when I go to town. Help me remember to ask You what I am forgetting before I head back to the house. Thank You. I praise You that You answer prayer. Thank You for talking to me about little and big things, important things and not so important things.

Abba, I do not even know where to begin. So help me, Holy Spirit, to think back. Help me go where I do not dare to trod alone. Go back in my memory and help me handle the pain there. I pray in Your Holy Spirit's power it will not hurt to go there now. I ask in the Mighty Name of my Jesus that

You will calm my fears, so I can even think about it, and write about it, and be able to talk about it.

What am I so afraid of? And how long have I been so afraid and what has calmed my fears within and without? I ask You, dear LORD Jesus, to calm my fears of even putting it down on paper. Handle my fear with faith, love and courage.

Abba, where are You going with this? What do I write and what do I not write? In 2008 during spring break of school I started asking if You wanted me to write about what You, God, had and were doing in my life. You let me know very clearly that was what You wanted me to do. I ask for a few simple words and the best words and give us listening ears.

I leave it in Your hands that You, God, will guide people as they need to read this book. It is to Your glory and honor and praise that I write it. It has been good for me, and I pray it will be good for those who read it, too. Help them gently understand a little of the world of mental illness, but above all let them come to an understanding they need You right now in their lives. Help them not wait until something awful happens in their lives to need You, for You and I both know they need You, God, now! Please touch lives through these words and Father save people for eternity. I love You and my heart breaks for people that do not know You in a close personal relationship. They just do not know, they just cannot comprehend what they are missing. It is not just missing Hell; there is so much more to You than just "fire insurance." You want to love us now. You want us to have abundant life now. You are never boring. You are never monotonous. I praise You and I thank You. In Jesus Name above all names, Amen.

(4)

If I Say Three Words, I Want People to Know Whether to Listen to Me or Not.

*A*bba Father, in 2008 I placed a fleece before You. I did not tell anyone what it was until after the fact. My gold colored mechanical pencil was lost. I prayed if You wanted me to write my story down, You would show me where it was. You have not only showed me once, but over and over again You showed me where it was each time I lost it again. Amy, Kristi, Crystal and Lorraine encouraged me to write it down. Cindy encouraged me to write it down, and that if I wrote for the right reasons—nothing was off limits. So I ask You—is it just between You and me? Do I just burn the pages as I write? Do I black out the names? Do I write it all? It is no longer a question of do I write, but what do I write? When do I write? Is it just for me? Or is it to help someone else? I ask in the Blessed and Precious Name of my Jesus, Amen.

I wore out that gold mechanical pencil. You, God, showed me I was to write with whatever I had, even if it was a Sharpie.

I do not do crafts at home as much as I did at one time. I get the crafts together for the three year olds for Sunday school at church where I am one of the teachers. I scrapbook by doing "faithbooking." It is a way of journaling life experiences and adding scripture to scrapbooks. I journal some, mostly just prayers and answers to prayers, but for the past year I have not been able to write except just short prayers. But I have put most of my effort into writing this book. I am bipolar. That means I have highs called manic and lows called depression, and sometimes I am very level. God has always led me through it, but it has been a journey with Him. It has been a process—a walk with Him from either depression or manic back to a sound mind and the mind of Christ. Would you allow God to lead you back to a right mind and the mind of Christ?

This book is no joy ride, but manic-depression is a roller coaster ride through life. It is up and down—over and over again. I have been out of the State hospital since spring of 2002, but during spring break of 2008, the medicine became ineffective so I had to come off it, and at the same time go on another medicine. We tried to do it this time without me having to go to the State hospital. I did it with the full support of my church behind me. They have prayed for me and encouraged me to keep talking this time. This time I have tried to stay very verbal. Even to the point of writing down things in the form of this book. It has been very healing for me to write. I see Dr. Greer as my family physician and Dr. Tom talks to me and explains things to me. I have Dr. Snowden as my psychologist, Dr.Wieck as my psychiatrist, and Bro. Randy and Pam, my pastor and his wife as my godly counsel. I have probably had more counsel out of the hospital this time than when I was in the hospitals in my past. I have continued to function this time, and I have begun to really live life. I do not know what the future holds, but Jesus holds my future, and He either carries me or walks with me back to a right mind, the mind of Christ. I praise Him that I am even alive. God gets all the glory and all the praise. As I look back over the time it took me to write this book, it has been a good time. It has been a time of healing, I pray it will be a time of healing for you as you read the book.

But as it is written:

"Eye has not seen, nor ear heard, Nor have entered into the heart of man The things which God has prepared for those who love Him." But God has revealed them to us through His Spirit. For the spirit searches all things, yes, the deep things of God. For what man knows the things of a man except the spirit of the man which is in him? Even so no one knows the things of God except the Spirit of God. Now we have received, not the spirit of the world, but the Spirit who is from God, that we might know the things that have been freely given to us by God. These things we also speak, not in words which man's wisdom teaches but which the Holy Spirit teaches, comparing spiritual things with spiritual. But the natural man does not receive the things of the Spirit of God, for they are foolishness to him; nor can he know them, because they are spiritually discerned. But he who is spiritual judges all things, yet he himself is rightly judged by no one. For "who has known the mind of the LORD that he may instruct Him?" But we have the mind of Christ. 1 Corinthians 2:9-16 (NKJV)

I Open the Door

❧

I was born in north central Texas. Innocently enough, my big brother, Dewayne said about me when I was little, "She can't talk." Did it become a part of me or is there some reason I do not talk much? I do not know. I have been afraid to talk since I was very, very little. I kept it all inside, conversations going on in my head, all bottled up that I would not tell anyone. I do not know why. In the Bible it talks about Mary, the mother of Jesus, that she pondered things—that she kept these things in her heart. Is that where these things are stored in me? Because my memory is not too good is it stored in my heart? My heart hurts, it physically hurts. My heart hurts for other people going through the same struggles I go through, but without any godly counsel, without God even. My heart hurts for people who are alone without Jesus to help them through this world. So invite Him into your heart right now before we go on with this journey together. Jesus will forgive you for anything except not asking for forgiveness and for Him to be your Savior in the first place. Trust Him now before it is too late. Do not put it off one more second. Just ask Him to come into your life for good and not for evil to give you a purpose and a plan for a future and a hope. God is good. He is good. God is faithful. Believe "my sin is my sin." Do not defend yourself and do not try to hide your sin. God sees you as you are and that is okay. God forgives. In Jesus name we have to ask.

March Friday PM 3-14-08

I remember Vacation Bible School as a very small child. Momma was the teacher in another class. I was not even in school yet. It was stormy and thundering that day. I reached my finger into the turtle's box, and he latched on to my finger and would not let go. Momma heard my screams and knew it was me. They got it off, but turtles do not let go even when it thunders. It was just a baby turtle, but then my finger was just a baby's too. I lift up empty hands to You, God. There is no scar, and I do not even know what finger that little turtle latched onto. Why then is it still an open wound in my heart? I got hurt at church. My finger is healed. I am okay now. Can memories hurt? Yes they can and they do. I bring You, Abba, Father my fingers. I do not even remember which one so I bring them all to You, for healing. I bring You my mind. I bring You my heart. I remember the memory of it frequently—when I see the turtles that wander into our yard and during VBS each year that I help I remember it. The memory still hurts; there is still an open wound there. I give it to You, God. Please make it better. Heal the hurt. Such a little thing—why does it take a whole page in this book? Why did it have its own room in my heart or was it in my head? I have got lots of rooms. Rooms I am afraid to go in—alone. I do not want to go in them without You, God. I called them dungeons when I was praying to You, Abba.

We moved a lot because of Daddy's job, which was road construction. But when my oldest brother started the second grade we settled in the town in Texas where Momma had gone to high school. Daddy worked away from home and was gone all week, but we stayed put. My grandparents on Momma's side of the family lived there too, as did my Uncle Eddie, Momma's brother and his wife, Aunt Nedra.

I did not make friends easily at school. I spent time against the wall during recess in elementary school. I was not in trouble; I just did not know how to belong with the other kids. I remember spending a lot of time in the bathroom during homeroom my sixth grade year of junior high. I felt sick each morning I had to go to school. I had a hard time adjusting to having to change rooms and going to different teachers.

Jesus answered and said to him,…For God so loved the world that He gave His only begotten Son, that whoever believes in Him should not perish but have everlasting life. For God did not send His Son into the world to condemn the world, but that the world through Him might be saved. John 3:10A and 16-17 (NKJV)

Then God said, "Let Us make man in Our image, according to Our likeness; let them have dominion over the fish of the sea, over the birds of the air, and over the cattle, over all the earth and over every creeping thing that creeps on the earth." So God created man in His own image; in the image of God He created him; male and female He created them. Genesis 1:26-27 (NKJV)

In the beginning was the Word, and the Word was with God, and the Word was God. He was in the beginning with God. All things were made through Him, and without Him nothing was made that was made. John 1:1-3 (NKJV)

And the Word became flesh and dwelt among us, and we beheld His glory, the glory as of the only begotten of the Father, full of grace and truth. John 1:14 (NKJV)

I do not remember who, but one of my pastors told me once that the Word is a name of Jesus so if we substitute Jesus' name for the Word in these verses, then this is what it says:

In the beginning was Jesus, and Jesus was with God, and Jesus was God. All things were made through Him, and without Him nothing was made that was made. And Jesus became flesh and dwelt among us, and we beheld His glory, the glory as of the only begotten of the Father, full of grace and truth.

Yours is the mighty power and glory and victory and majesty. Everything in the heavens and earth is yours, O Lord, and this is your kingdom. We adore you as being in control of everything. Riches and honor come from you alone, and you are the Ruler of all mankind; your hand controls power and might, and it is at your discretion that men are made great and given strength. O our God, we thank you and praise your glorious name. 1 Chronicles 29:11-13 (The Living Bible)

March Saturday 3-15-08

Abba, Immanuel means God with us. Have You always been with me? Even as a child? As a child I got locked out of the house once. Even then I learned there were some places I was not allowed and did not belong. And home was one of those places. It made an impact on me. They were inside, and I was outside. I open the door for You LORD Jesus. Why did it make such an impact on me? Why did I even care? I just remember somehow it hurt me. Hurt me inside. Can you heal the hurt in me, LORD Jesus? Abba, Father, please come into these rooms I have kept closed for so long. I will go into it only with You, Abba and Jesus and the Holy Spirit. I want a majority with me when I go in them. I was a little girl; a little girl who thought she belonged until then. Then she did not belong anywhere.

Abba, thank You God, for Your God-vacuum. Thank You for times in my life when I was so empty—until I came to You, LORD. Why did it take me so long to come to You? Please forgive Momma and Daddy; they did not even know what they did. I forgive them. In Jesus Mighty Name I ask, Amen.

March Saturday 3-1-2008

Abba, Father, I just do not know where to begin. Why? Why did I not know that Jesus loved me as a little child and teenager? I went to church. I went to Vacation Bible School. I was in GA's; I was even in the youth choir at church. But it never sunk in that You, Jesus, loved me.

Abba, when I was a little girl, I thought You, God, were like an ogre. I did not know that we are made in Your image. Abba, I did not get the part at all that God became flesh and dwelt among us.

Jesus, You found out by experience what it is like to be one of us. God, blow my mind with Your Word. Blow my mind with Your glory and majesty. I have been afraid to ask that—always I have put a limitation on what I would allow You to do in my life. I am taking all control away from me. Jehovah, do in my life, in my heart, mind, will, emotions, body, soul and spirit—what You have always wanted to do for me right from the very beginning. I fear You—I respect You—I am in awe of You. I am willing now to do it Your way. And I open the doors to You at least all I can; doors in my heart and doors in my mind—some locked from the inside and some locked from the outside. I do not even know how to get into them. I only know I do not want to go into them alone. I need You to go in them with me because You hold the keys. I need You to be God. I need You to be in control. That is what I am learning in the Crown Financial Bible Study. Abba, I am asking, "Do You want me to go through these doors? Is it necessary? Do I have to? Could we just do this in heaven where it will be safe?" I ask in Jesus Name, Amen.

(6)

What Happens When it is Quiet?

God spoke to me:

"What happens to the candy when you make hot spiced tea?"

I told Him: "It is just a hard piece of cinnamon fire stick candy—I put it in a cup of cold water and put it in the microwave. I heat it on HIGH for two minutes and when it is soft—I stretch it out on the bottom of the cup. I use a spoon and make the candy spread out so it will dissolve and become a part of the liquid. I stir it till it is completely dissolved. Then I add the spiced tea mix."

God spoke to me:

"That is what I want to do to you—Stretch you out."

I told Him: "Then stretch me out, LORD God. You do it with my full cooperation. You are God, and I am not and I place my crown at Your feet.

Jesus blood was shed at Calvary. It is not saved in a quart jar. It was applied to the altar in heaven where it still forgives our sins today. It is enough. It will always be enough. It will not run out. It will not go bad. Jesus saves. Forever, Jesus saves.

I have been allowed to talk before my church twice two years ago during the service. I praise God for the opportunities for several reasons. I wanted to tell them what God had done behind the scenes because they prayed for me. I wanted to have a chance to thank them for their prayers. God told me He did not care if I stood before them with fear and trembling I was to tell them my testimony. A testimony is where you tell what God has done in your life.

Some of you reading this book have known me for a long time. Some of you have prayed for me a long time. I have wanted an opportunity to be able to thank you for your prayer support over the years. Thank you for allowing me to do so today. Your prayers moved God to work behind the scenes of what you and I were able to see with our physical eyes. God answered your prayers even and especially during times, even for months, when I could not pray myself. I thank each of you and I thank and praise my God.

Some of you do not know me. Whether you know me or not, my testimony is unknown to most of you because I have kept silent. I do not want to be silent anymore. I want people to know what God has done in my life.

There is a song that says: Count your blessings, name them one by one. And it will surprise you what the LORD has done. By Johnson Oatman Jr.

Blessings from God do not always look like blessings to us. Most people do not take pictures of the bad things that happen in our lives. We do not pull out a scrapbook of a divorce and ask others to look at it. Today I am asking you to look at some bad things that happened in my life that some may not call blessings, but God has worked them for good.

(7)

I Remember

🌹

Written Christmas season 2004

"*I* remember Christmas at Grandmother Mabel and Granddaddy Corky's when I was growing up. All my aunts and uncles and their families would come: Uncle Eddie and Aunt Nedra; Aunt Wanda and Uncle Kyle; Uncle R G and Aunt Estie; Uncle Hoyt and Aunt Mary. Uncle James, Aunt Teddie, Meredith, their son, and Jackie their daughter, who was my age, would come and sometimes I would get to go home with them. And of course Momma, Daddy, and Dewayne (my older brother) and Bryan (my younger brother) were there, too.

And we would go to Grandmother Zay's house and all of my Daddy's side of the family would gather at her house: Uncle Kenneth and Aunt Sue with Dale and Steve; Uncle Bill and Kelena, Billy Wayne and Tanya were there.

And we would go to Dr. Bill's house and my Granddad's side of the family would gather there: Uncle Orion and Aunt Dutch; Aunt Jewel, Butch, Cindy, Mildred and Camille; Uncle Dick and Aunt Bob; Aunt Minnie; Aunt Pearl and Dr. Bill; Uncle Luther and Aunt Ellen; Uncle Herbert and Aunt Gladis. That is what made it special—the people who were there. It was not the gifts, although we got some. It was the laughter and the love.

Some years, Aunt Wanda, (Momma's sister), and Uncle Kyle could not be there because they were in Japan while they were stationed there in the Air Force. I remember listening to a tape they sent one year. We cried when we heard it. How we missed them!

And then there was the Christmas that Eddie Claude died. He was Uncle Eddie's, (Momma's brother) and Aunt Nedra's baby boy. Jackie and I were in the guest room when they came from the hospital and told us. It was the saddest Christmas Day ever. How I loved to hold Eddie Claude when he was a baby. He died before he was a year and a half old.

I remember there was a huge solid door, about eight inches thick that opened to the freezer at the frozen food locker plant that my Granddad Corky owned and where Momma worked. My brothers and I worked there too while we were growing up. I did not like going in that freezer—I was always afraid my brothers would hold the door shut and I would not be able to get out, and I would freeze to death. You know what? They never did, so why was I so afraid?

Mama says I was saved as a little girl. When I was just a child, I went down during the invitation and prayed with Bro. Kenneth. But he prayed so fast, I could not keep up with him. Everybody thought I was saved. I was baptized. I remember I choked on the water when he brought me up out of the water when I was baptized. I remember there was no change in my life. I tried to read the Bible, but it never made any sense to me. And my prayers consisted of "Help me pass this test" even though I had not even studied the night before the test. As a young teenager I read in the Bible, the Ten Commandments, and I thought to myself that I never had done any of those things.

I remember stealing something from the grocery store, and Momma making me take it back. It was not to be the last time I stole.

Thou shalt not steal. Exodus 20:15 (NKJV)

During my childhood and teenage years, I would rededicate my life to Christ, but there was no change in my life in how I acted when I got back home. I read the Bible some, but I did not understand it. I read God's Ten Commandments. I told God I had not ever broken any of them. I soon discovered by the time I was an adult, I had broken almost every one of the Ten Commandments. God showed me I needed Him. I needed His forgiveness, but I could not accept that Jesus Christ's forgiveness was enough to save me.

In high school I became addicted to pornography. I would read it; feel so dirty and guilty that I would throw it away. But I would go back and find more over and over again. When I could not find any more pornography that led to having sex with my boyfriend, Buh.

For this is the will of God, your sanctification: that you should abstain from sexual immorality; 1 Thessalonians 4:3 (NKJV)

I started drinking alcohol. I prayed to have a baby. I was not even married yet. But I became pregnant. Then I asked Buh if he wanted to abort her. It does not make any sense does it, to ask God for a baby and then not accept her. Roe versus Wade had just passed. I am so glad Buh said, "No!"

That I remember at all is such a miracle to me, because I had 21 electric shock treatments during a time while I was depressed. I could not remember anything at all. It wiped out my complete memory. Momma had to introduce me to my own son, Jay. The memories came back, but the bad memories came back first. I do not recommend electric shock treatments to anyone. Sights, sounds, smells and tastes will trigger a memory to flood back into my mind. It is kind of overwhelming.

Buh and I married. I quit going to church when I became pregnant first, and then I married. I felt dirty. I felt so dirty the day I married. I had a church wedding, I had on the white dress, and Daddy walked me down the aisle. But I was dirty. Sin does that to you. I always felt shameful and dirty and guilty every time my husband and I had sex after that even after Buh and I married. I did not think God could forgive me, not of that. So I did not go to church, and I quit seeing my friends from church. I quit singing the Christian songs I loved, and I quit praying for a long, long, long time. Sin does that. Sin separates us from God sometimes for a very long time. But I learned later God forgives when we ask in repentance for our sins. I just would not ask. We have to believe He can forgive anything and everything, because He will.

Remember the Sabbath and keep it holy. Exodus 20:8A (NKJV)

Buh had graduated from high school in his home town a year before me. I continued my senior year of high school pregnant. I was one of the first girls allowed to continue schooling pregnant. I loved being pregnant. I loved the new clothes. I felt better than I ever had before. I loved feeling Jen kicking me. Because Jen was due before school was out, I had to turn in my senior theme early, before the others in the class. Nanny, Buh's Mom, typed it for me. It was on pregnancy. I received a good grade on it, but it did not prepare me for the pain of having Jen, or for being a good mother to her. Buh went to college during the week and was home with me at Momma and Daddy's house during the weekends. Buh and I moved into an apartment by the time Jen was ready to be born.

I remember I kept tensing up during labor every time I had a contraction. I remember Buh smelled like smoke, and it upset my stomach so he could not be in the room with me during labor. I kept saying to Momma, "It hurts" and Momma kept saying to me, "I know." Dr. Greer was at a circus when Jen decided to come. But he arrived in time to bring her into this world. I remember when they put Jen on my stomach after she was born, she felt so warm, so much like she belonged there, that I quit trembling while she was there. But then they took her away. It did not matter how many warm blankets they piled on me, I still shook. Buh spent the night in my hospital room with me. I did not get to see Jen again until the next day

Jen was a Daddy's girl. She bonded with Buh from the very beginning. How he could make her laugh, giggle, smile and coo. He was a wonderful Daddy!

I went back to classes at high school and Momma kept Jen. I do not know what I would have done without her. I graduated about a month after Jen was born.

Summer started and Buh was out of college for the semester. Buh worked for a feed and grain elevator. At first he mixed grain and loaded out feed orders. Later during wheat harvest he started driving an 18 wheeler truck hauling grain to the elevators in Saginaw, Texas. Jen and I would go with him sometimes.

I do not remember as many details about this night. During that summer there were many trips to the elevators to deliver wheat to the grain bins there. Many a night I would watch as the trailer of the 18 wheeler would get full, and I would motion for Buh to pull up until that section would get full and again and again till the whole trailer was full. Then Buh would tarp it down and we would go to the elevator to deliver it. It was long hours, all night and all day back and forth. God's divine hand was on us all the time that we were driving. We were too ignorant of how much God loved us that we did not even know He was keeping us on the road when Buh's eyes could not keep open any more or just when open eyes were glazed over and could not see the road ahead, yet we drove on. I praise You, God.

When I started writing this, I was remembering one night in particular. I do not remember why I was on top of the trailer. I just remember falling off between the trailer and the truck. I remember Buh's hand grabbing mine and pulling me back up before I fell on the truck's platform.

I did not know how to be a good mother to my kids or a good wife to Buh. But I was not looking in the right place for the answers to life's problems. I did not read the Bible, and if I ever prayed I do not remember it. Jesus loved me was so foreign to me. Why did I not know that Jesus loved me? I thought God was an ogre, ugly and too big to grasp a hold of, when all along He was trying to grasp me. He was showing me in ways only now I am beginning to see that He loves us very much. That He loved even me. Beautiful beyond description that is what God is. And big—my God left heaven for a time as Jesus and became a tiny baby, defenseless except for a Momma and a Daddy who loved Him. My God became poor so He would know what it was like for us. My God died—Jesus died so we could really live. Forgiveness, peace, joy, abundant life that all begins the second we trust and believe in Him. Thru the trials, temptations and triumphs God is very much with us. Thank You God for grabbing hold of my hand.

We moved to east Texas. Buh continued to go to college and worked at a liquor store the rest of the time. I stayed home with Jen. I did not know what to do after high school. Going to school is all I had ever remembered doing. But I was not about to go to college with all those people I did not know, even though Momma and Daddy said they would pay my way. I was scared of people I did not know, and this world was full of them.

Buh took flying lessons while he was in college. I spent the day before we flew to Nanny's smoking a ham in the old refrigerator smoker that Mr. Nixon showed Buh how to build. It was Easter weekend, and I was furnishing the ham for lunch at Nanny's. The next morning I mixed up bread for it to rise on the way to Nanny's. It was windy, but I pleaded with Buh to fly us to Nanny's. Buh was a student pilot, and we used his trainer's Cessna to fly that day. Jen was not even strapped in. She was in the back throwing up it was so bumpy. I remember thinking this is what it is like to die. We touched down on a small runway, but immediately the wind picked us back up into the air and put us back down on a plowed field right beside the runway. We continued down the field until the tricycle wheel of the plane buried into the plowed ground and the plane balanced, it seemed a long time, on its nose before flipping upside down. Everything from the back went forward including Jen. Buh released his seat belt and turned to catch her in mid air before she hit the windshield. I was upside down in the plane still strapped in. Everything was backwards, and it took me a while to figure out how to release the seat belt and fall to the top of the plane which now was underneath me. If I had died that day, I would have gone to hell. Jay would have never been born.

I called my family and told them about the crash. Uncle Kyle had flown to my Grandparents' house and he told us we needed to fly home that day. He said it was like getting back on a horse when you had been bucked off. So Uncle Kyle flew us home that evening. Thank You, God, I would not have flown to Australia, Boston, Okinawa or St. Louis later in my life if we had not flown back home that day. I praise You. I did not then, but I do now. I give You all the glory and all the praise. I ask it in the Precious Name of my Jesus, Amen.

I worked at Red Coleman's in the Deli making sandwiches and as a cashier for a while. It was not the same store as where Buh worked; it was the convenience store part of the block. I followed the crowd most of my growing up years and even after I was married and had children. I did not ask God how I was to live my life for most of my life even while I was a Christian. I let my friends tell me what to do, and some of those friends turned out to be not so friendly. I missed out on God all those years, and I will never get them back. Sins of bad decisions, bad choices, I turned my back on God. I thought I could run my life just fine. I was wrong.

Then I started working for Mac at his greenhouse. I watered, fertilized, potted plants and took cuttings—I mean that in a bad way. In that I stole cuttings and took them home and started plants. Mac was the nicest man to work for, but I stole from him. I later paid him back for what I stole from him and he forgave me.

Thou shalt not steal Exodus 20:15 (NKJV)

God brought it home to me again—I had sinned against God. Mac taught me to pray—everyday he would go to town and get us a hamburger from the Sonic, and he always prayed before we ate together. We would sit on a swing that was under a huge tree by a pond at the back of the greenhouses and we would pray before we ate. Such a simple thing, but it would have a lifelong influence on me. They asked me, but I would not go to church with them.

When I was depressed during my marriage my husband tried to get me to go see a doctor but I would not. I would not have sex with my husband very often because I always felt so dirty and guilty because of my sin. One day Buh put his foot down and gave me an ultimatum. Either I would have sex with him or he was going to find someone else. I gave him permission to go find someone else. I am so sorry for those decisions.

I have been falling down, throwing up drunk. I drank socially, usually not to get drunk just to take the edge off life. I do not drink beer or alcohol anymore; I praise You God for that. But I do not look at beer signs very long, I do not look at the bottles, and I do not watch the advertisements on TV. I do not want to go back to that lifestyle. I made the worst decisions in my life while under the influence of alcohol. It felt good for a while, but then I would wake up to the consequences of the decisions made and what I had done while I was drunk. Many times Jen was not being taken care of while we were partying, and she was not big enough to take care of herself.

Jen was little when my friends took me Christmas shopping. My husband gave me the money to buy gifts. I used most of the money on me. When I bought groceries while I was married it was what I wanted, I did not care about what my family liked. I would not learn to cook the foods they wanted.

I did not know how to handle money. Momma said "it burns a hole in your pocket." I just have to spend it. I robbed God. For years, while I was married, I did not go to church and I did not tithe.

I quit work at Mac's, and Jen and I went to stay at Pa and Nanny's house in north central Texas. They are my Father-in-law and Mother-in-law. Buh, my husband came to see us. I prayed for another baby. I only had sex with Buh that one time that summer, and I got pregnant with Jay. It amazes me that God answered my prayer. I was not going to church. I was not acknowledging God in any other way. But He listened and heard me when I asked Him. And God answered—Yes!

I went back to Buh, and when he graduated from East Texas State University, we moved farther east in Texas. Buh worked as a truck driver for a steel company. I stayed home and kept Jen. And I stole again, always more and bigger this time.

Thou shalt not steal. Exodus 20:15 (NKJV)

Nanny (my Mother-in-law) and Goo Goo (my Grandmother-in-law) came a few weeks before our baby was due to stay with Jen and me until he was ready to be born. Buh was on the truck and gone for days at a time. Nanny drove me over every bumpy road we could find trying to see if Jay would come. Nanny's days off from work were running out, and she needed to go back home. We walked the walking trail that was behind our apartments and that did not work. I was having false labor but not the real thing. I would go to the hospital, and they would send me home. We had the best times, we ate out and we ate in. We visited and laughed. Finally on April 9, I went to see my doctor at his office, and he said it was time. Jay came a little after midnight so that his birthday falls on April 10, one year after Terrible Tuesday, which is what they called the tornado that hit Wichita Falls, Texas in 1979.

I called Momma, and she came to stay with us so Nanny and Goo Goo could go home. I was not nice to Mama. I was not even civil to Momma. I would not let her be with Jay. God showed me how cruel I could be without Him in my life. But I just went on with my life as if nothing had ever happened. I was mean, hateful and spiteful to her. I do not even know why.

But I took all my hate out on her. She left and cried all the way home. I broke her heart.

Honor thy Father and Mother that your days may be long upon the land which the LORD your God is giving you. Exodus 20:12 (NKJV)

I was unloving to Momma for years upon years. I do not even know why. I was unloving to a lot of people. I did not care to put out the effort it took to love them. Some of them really did love me, and I just did not care. I am never more unlike God than when I am unloving to the people who surround me. God is not here in person for us to love Him. He has placed people in my life for me to show Him how much I love Him by how much I love them. Some people are easier to love than others, but we are called to love them all.

Buh and I decided to build a house out in the country in east Texas. That was what I had always wanted. I was allowed to choose the house plan and to pick out exactly how I wanted it to be and what went into it. Jen started to the school there even before we finished building the house. I would drive her to the house, so she could meet the school bus. I would stay to see how things were progressing on the house until she came home from school in the afternoon. Then we would go back to the apartment. I moved stuff in the car out to the new house little by little each day.

Momma and Daddy came to visit when we moved into the new house. Why she forgave me—I will never know. Daddy helped us with the driveway while they were there.

Buh's family all came for Christmas to our house that year. I loved having the house full of people.

But I was afraid to be alone in the house at night when Buh was gone on the truck for days at a time. I could manage it during the day when it was light outside. Afraid does not even describe it. Fear overwhelmed me. I was so afraid that one night when one of the children came to my door crying, I would not let him in. I was afraid to get out of the bed in the dark. The next morning after it became light I found him asleep in the hall where he had cried himself to sleep.

Then Buh was laid off from his trucking job. I stood in the kitchen and cried the day the people came to look at the house to buy it. They were the only ones to whom I had to show it because they bought it.

Buh got a job in Fort Worth working for a finance company. We moved in with my Uncle Kyle and Aunt Wanda, (Momma's sister) and their daughter, Jana and son, Ken. They let us live there while we looked for a place to live. We had the best time. I went to church with my Aunt a few times. We finally bought a trailer house to live in, and we stayed in a trailer park close to my Aunt's house.

We were married with two children when Buh was transferred to east Texas. So we moved the trailer house there. I was still shy and did not make friends easily. God used my loneliness to create a need for Him. I desperately needed someone to love me. We had moved five times. I was lost. I was alone, even in a crowd. I never felt I belonged. One day I was watching PTL again on TV, and after it was over I got down on my knees and asked Jesus into my heart to save me. I started going to church at a Baptist church close to where we lived in the trailer park. I joined the church by saying that I had been saved as a child, I did not say anything about the fact that I had just been saved at home.

I attended Sunday mornings and nights and Wednesday nights at the church near us and went to their Baptist Women's which met during the week; they were going through the Experiencing God Bible study. I was babysitting at the time, and when I went to Baptist Women's, they let me bring my children and my baby sitting children to stay in the nursery. I worked sometimes on Sundays in the nursery to make up for it. I was finally growing in the LORD. That is when I started seeing a positive change in my life. I started reading the Bible and understood it. I started praying. Then I started praying and fasting on weekends for God to save my husband and heal my marriage. Then Buh walked in the trailer one day, he said that he did not want to live with me anymore, and told me he was leaving and he wanted a divorce, he had good reasons to leave. I said these words to my husband, "I wish I could have sex with him." I was referring to another man besides my husband. That is the moment my husband left me, not that day but before the week was over he was gone. I told you he had good reason to leave me. I hurt him deeply that day. I have asked him to forgive me. He said I was the one that needed to forgive him. I have forgiven my husband, but there are people in my family who have not.

It was just me and the children, Jen and Jay, in the trailer house in east Texas. Jay was about a year and a half old and Jen was about six. For the first time in my life I was all on my own. I had been fasting for the healing of my marriage for a couple of months every weekend. I intensified my fasting and started going without water. I went to church Sunday morning, but did not go Sunday night. I did not tell anyone my husband had left me. I did not know what to do except pray. I started reading my Bible, and I started taking things out of context. I sent Jen and Jay next door to eat with our neighbors that night.

I was not prepared for what came next. During that same weekend I had my first full blown manic episode. I was convinced the rapture had happened and that I had been left behind. I not only lost Buh that week, but Satan convinced me that Jesus had come back and I had been left behind. How would that have affected you? It devastated me! I lost all hope. I did not know what to do. I was so scared. I did not know whom to trust because anyone that came into contact with me had been "left behind" also. To those of you who do not know what the rapture is; some day Jesus is coming back to get His church of believers and take them to Heaven and those who do not have a relationship with Jesus will be left behind. We are to be ready for when that happens. But I believed the rapture had happened, and I was left behind. I did not trust anyone, and I was not talking or listening to anyone.

I got Jen up Monday morning and sent her to school. The children I baby sat came that morning, but one of the Moms saw that there was something wrong with me. She got in touch with my husband at work. He made arrangements for Nanny to meet us halfway between where we lived. By then I did not trust anyone. If they were still there, to me that meant they had been left behind also. I did not trust God because He had left me behind. It did not really happen, but I believed it had. I would not read the book of Revelation in the Bible for years to come.

No Buh, God did not answer my prayer, He did not heal my marriage. That is what I thought at the time. God answered— He answered no. It just was not the answer I wanted to hear.

And no Jesus.

That is what I thought at the time.

Nanny was still there. Michael was still there. I did not trust anybody. I started eating and drinking fluids again. Momma found out I was at Nanny's a few days later, and she was the one who got me into a mental hospital in north central Texas. Momma was still there. I did not talk to anyone, not even my psychiatrist. My psychiatrist would not say anything. He just sat in my room waiting for me to speak. But I was so troubled, I would not talk. I was a fairly new Christian only a few months old. My church family, my support, was gone. To me I did not have my husband anymore, and I did not think I had Jesus anymore either. I called my pastor in east Texas while I was in Red River Hospital. He told me they were praying for me. They were still there.

I was not left behind, the rapture has not really happened, yet. Abba, You speak to me at times when I am alone telling me that You will never leave me nor forsake me. Why is it still fresh? Why does it still hurt? Will You heal me? Will You make it better?

God gently began teaching me to trust Him again.

For God so loved the world that He gave His only begotten Son, that whoever believes in Him should not perish but have everlasting life. John 3:16 (NKJV)

I got out of the hospital; I was not well even after a couple of months of therapy and counseling. Why? Because I still was not talking about what had happened. Everyone assumed I was depressed over my husband leaving me. I still could not talk to anyone about believing I had been left behind.

*****

Jesus is the cornerstone.

The stone which the builders rejected Has become the chief cornerstone. This was the LORD's doing; It is marvelous in our eyes. This is the day the LORD has made; We will rejoice and be glad in it. Psalm 118:22-24 (NKJV)

Jesus said to them, "Have you never read in the Scriptures: 'The stone which the builders rejected Has become the chief cornerstone. This was the LORD's doing, And it is marvelous in our eyes'? Matthew 21:42 (NKJV)

Jesus is speaking "Have you not even read this Scripture: 'The stone which the builders rejected Has become the chief cornerstone. This was the LORD's doing, And it is marvelous in our eyes'?" Mark 12:10-11 (NKJV)

*****

God understands rejection the most because He went through it. Jesus was rejected to death.

*****

Jesus is the cornerstone. That is the foundation on which we build; He is over us and under us and can be in us if we will only allow it and ask Him in, but He does not force Himself upon us. Jesus will never leave me nor forsake me. He did not leave me then—He carried me the whole time in his arms.

And in the wilderness where you saw how the LORD your God carried you, as a man carries his son, in all the way that you went until you came to this place.
Deuteronomy 1:31 (NKJV)

I would get over the depression and get better. I would praise God that I had been healed, and I would stop taking my medication. Then I would cycle again; I would go back into depression. The doctor at the hospital only saw my depression side each time. And that is how they diagnosed me—major depression. It would be over ten years before they really knew what was wrong with me—manic depression also known as bipolar disorder. Up and down. It was a roller coaster ride. Over the years I have been in Wichita General twice on the psychiatric floor. I had electric shock treatments. That I remember at all is a blessing from God, and I praise Him for the good and the bad memories. Momma spent years teaching me names to faces and places and dates and events. I still have trouble with them. My Momma has stood by me in all of this. When anyone else would have walked away and given up, she did not. When I was little, my big brother would say about me, "She can't talk." My Momma was there when I truly could not talk for myself. She spoke for me, she told them I was not faking and that I really was not like the way I was acting. I Praise God.

I cannot get any more stupid than not knowing: not knowing names of anyone, not even my own preschool son's name, not knowing people and places and events. But that is the point I came to after I had electric shock treatments over a span of several years. I do not recommend it to anyone because the bad memories come back first and that was what I wanted to forget.

I moved in with Nanny and Pa after I was released from the hospital. Nanny and Pa taught me about unconditional love. They have always loved me, even when I was divorced from their son. God said, "**Let him go.**" Even though I did not want a divorce, I obeyed God. My parents-in-law still let me and Jay live with them. They did not owe me anything, but they let me and Jay live with them. I started going back to church at the Baptist church and sometimes at the Assembly of God. Nanny, my mother-in-law, was a new Christian too and so was Michael, my brother-in-law. It was special growing together in the LORD. I was baptized again because I wanted people to know I had been saved when I asked Jesus into my heart in the trailer house before I left east Texas.

I visited at the church where Momma and Daddy went and that Sunday. Bro. Ted, the pastor, had us get down on our knees to pray. I decided that day that is where I wanted to go to church. So Jay and I moved back to the town where I grew up and lived with Momma and Daddy and started going to church with them. Jen stayed with her dad because I did not want her to have to change schools again.

Daddy worked close to home now and came home every night after work. We all went to church where Bro. Ted was pastor. He taught me to get down on my knees before Holy God. I do not know how many times "I went down to the front" at church; it was too many times to number. I was baptized again. I just did not feel saved. I even surrendered my life to special service. I doubted my salvation. If things did not go the way I thought they should and God did not answer my prayers the way I thought He should, I would think I was lost, that I was not saved, and I walked the aisle so many times I lost count. I was baptized three times.

I think I was sin sick. I was not being specific when I confessed my sins to God. I would just ask Him to forgive all my sins but never pin pointed a specific sin so that I could confess it and repent of it and turn away from that particular sin. Now I get quiet and ask God what my sin is. He already knows what it is, but He has to let me know what it is so I repent and not do those sins anymore. So I get specific now when I ask for forgiveness.

I get depressed like clockwork on a rotating schedule. Sometimes I am up and sometimes I am down; sometimes I am level and as close to normal as I can be. How much is caused by sin, unconfessed sin? What I call sin sick. How much is just how God created me in the first place? I do not know, but I have learned I better deal with the sin issue in my life.

God says choose joy. It may not feel good while I am going through it, but I can choose joy. I can praise God in the process and be thankful it will not always be like this—not here on earth but especially not when I go to heaven. In heaven there will not be even a hint or shadow of depression or manic. I praise God and thank Him for that. And we are not here on earth but a fraction of a billi-second compared to how long we will be in heaven.

Abba, Thank You, Father, that Eddie Claude is in Heaven with You. Thank you that he is well. I do not know if people age in Heaven. I like to think Grandmother Mabel and Granddaddy Corky are holding him just like I used to. And he smiles and coos at them. Or maybe even better, he grew up in Heaven. Thank You either way, Father, I praise You.

Abba Father, please forgive me for asking Buh if he wanted to abort Jen. I thank You, God, that Buh said he wanted Jen. Buh wanted to marry me. Buh wanted God's baby that I had asked for. Thank You God for Buh and Jen. She is one of my most precious treasures I have here on earth.

Abba, I praise You that I am able to remember the good and the bad memories. Thank You.

Jesus, forgive me and thank You for forgiving me for having sex outside of marriage. Forgive me for not going to church as a young adult. Thank You for bringing me into Your family and into a relationship with all three of You—Abba, Jesus and Your

Holy Spirit. My life was so empty before I came to know You personally—three persons equal one God, the Holy Trinity. Thank You for forgiving me and working in me to bring me to this point today. I cannot imagine my life without You—it would not be living at all without all three of You.

Jesus, thank You for Your hand on Buh's when he caught me the night I fell off of the truck trailer. Thank You I did not get hurt. Thank You that in all that driving we did not hurt anyone else either. There were lots of miles that way. Lots of miles when Buh was by himself and You took care of him on the road and You took care of Jen and me and later on Jay, too.

Abba Father, I praise You. I thank You. It could have all ended that day of the plane crash so very differently. But we were okay, bruised a little, but very much alive. I do not know if I even thanked You then. I thank You now. I give You the credit. I praise You we are alive to tell the story.

Abba, I need You to guide me. I need You to lead me. I need You to control me: my actions, my reactions, my tongue and even my thoughts. Forgive me for following the crowd and living my life away from You. I cannot blame my actions and reactions on other people. It is my choice. Please forgive me for the times I have allowed other people to influence my choices and actions that resulted in sin against You. Thank You for forgiving me. I praise You, God.

Father, thank you for Mac and his wife Billie and the godly influence they had on my life. Thank You, Abba, that You listen and You answer prayer. I am so proud of You.

Abba, forgive me for not taking care of Jen. Forgive me for getting drunk. I praise You for deliverance in this area of my life. I see Your hand in it all. I praise You. There is victory in Jesus. Thank You.

Abba, I am sorry that I was so greedy with the money You gave me. I did not take into account what my family liked to eat. I only thought of me. I did not give You a tithe of my money either. It all belongs to You, and You allow us to have the money with the only request of 10% to go back to You, God, through the local church. I am sorry that I robbed You of the tithe money that was supposed to be Yours, LORD. All the time I was married I only thought of me and what I thought would make me happy. I had no regard for You, God. I never asked You anything. I just asked for what I wanted. I am so sorry. Please forgive me

Father, please forgive me, I hurt Momma so much. Not just then, but a whole lifetime of hurt. Cleanse me; I do not ever want to break her heart again. I am so sorry I hurt her like that. Please make things right between us. Teach me to love her like You love her, LORD, unconditionally. Thank You that now she is one of my best friends. Thank You for Momma.

Abba, forgive me for not even caring, much less not loving. I pray for Your love to flow through me. I want to love even those who may be very unloving to me and hard to love. I pray to love my Momma and Daddy. I pray to love my family, friends, the people I associate with, strangers and even my enemies. I pray for a love that does not come from me but from You. Fill me with the Holy Spirit and Your love. Thank You and I praise You. Thank You for taking away things and people in my life that led me to a relationship with You and my LORD Jesus. You are worth all the pain I went through. I glorify You.

God, I do not remember how long I was in the hospital before I got to go to the room where we did crafts, but I know, God, You met me there. Feeling worthless was one of the first things You started working with me about. I was in a mental hospital in north central Texas. I had just gone through, what I now know was, my first full blown manic episode. I felt worthless and betrayed by the two loves of my life, my husband and my Jesus. It was not true about You, Jesus, leaving me and You gradually started to convince me that that part of it was a lie. But I was devastated. I went into a major depression that lasted for years. I was over the manic stage and was in a deep depression. I felt like "junk" like I had been thrown away and discarded with the trash. I felt totally abandoned. The first thing, You, Abba and Jesus and the Holy Spirit did for me was to get me into the hands of people who cared and loved me and then into a mental hospital. They treated me with love and respect though I could not talk to them much. They started by meeting needs. They cooked the food I ate, they washed my clothes for me, they changed the linens on the bed and washed them, and then they provided crafts for me to do. The plaque I chose was a little piece of plaster to be painted. It had a rainbow on it and these words: "God don't make junk." Ethel Waters said it, and that was the start back up out of that deep dark abyss called depression and back to trusting God again. As I painted that little plaque, God, You started speaking to my heart that I was not junk to You. I did not have a Bible, just those words to hold to. It was a start to trusting You again.

Abba, those little words gave me Your hope that You had not given up on me. Thank You and I praise You for not giving up on me. I praise You and thank You, You never left my side and You provided a safe place for me to start the journey with You out of that deep dark pit of despair, of depression and back to a sound mind. Thank You that You gave me worth. Jesus, You thought enough of us to die for our sins. Forgive me for feeling worthless. You showed us how much we are worth to You when Jesus suffered and died on the cross to buy us back into Your kingdom. Thank You, that whosoever may can come and thank You that whosoever means me, too. It cost Jesus His life to pay the price necessary for us to become a member in Your family of God. Forgive me. Before I came to You, I was worthless, but God, You saw the difference Your Son could make in my life. Thank You, I am eternally grateful for You allowing me into Your kingdom.

Abba, please help Buh to know I am sorry for hurting him. Help me forgive him. Help him forgive me. Thank You for forgiving me. I pray You will forgive him. I pray my family will forgive him.

Jesus, I am sorry I rejected You for so long. I am sorry You had to endure the pain and suffering of beatings and scourging and carrying the cross and dying on the cross. Please forgive me.

I have been rejected too; it hurts when someone does not love you anymore and leaves. Thank You that no matter what I have done against You, even when I rejected You as I was growing up and as a young adult, You have never left me nor forsaken me. I may have thought at times You had, but You were right there with me all the time. As Bro. Jim says: "You God are closer than our very breath."

Thank You and I praise You for Your presence in my life. Forgive me for feeling rejected. You accepted me, chose me to be in Your family. It just does not get any better than that. You are the best DADDY I have ever had. You know how to love me by meeting my needs. One of those needs was just talking to someone. Thank You that You are always listening to me. Thank You for my counselors who listen and talk with me. Thank You for speaking through Your Word, the Bible, Your love letters to us. I am sorry that You, Jesus, were rejected by men. It is an awful feeling. Thank You that You, Jesus, are alive and at the right hand of God the Father, still interceding for us and with us by Your Holy Spirit at the same time. I praise You that You did not give up on me. Maybe I needed to know what this feels like so I can know just a little of what it felt like when You, Jesus were rejected. You never left me alone, not even and especially, when there was no one else in the room with me. You, God were there all along. God, You have never let me fall any further than my knees or to my face prostrate on the floor before You. You carry me, and I will not fall out of Your arms.

Abba, help me remember people's names. I put the wrong name on people and it is hard to get the right name to the right face. Thank You, Abba, for adopting me into Your family. Thank You for Momma who patiently taught me who was who in my family and church family. I thank You for every person who was so patient with me and for those who were not. Thank You for the good and the bad memories. I praise You. Thank You that I do not have to know it all because You know it all. I depend upon Your wisdom, Your knowledge, Your understanding, Your guidance and the mind of Christ.

Forgive me for feeling and being at times very stupid. Forgive me for making decisions based entirely on my way of thinking without seeking Your wisdom and guidance. Thank You when we ask for wisdom—wisdom is what You give us. I ask for Your wisdom, knowledge, understanding, revelation, sound judgment and discernment to grace my neck. I ask in Jesus Name and to Your glory, Amen.

(8)

The Armor of God

Finally, my brethren, be strong in the Lord and in the power of His might. Put on the whole armor of God, that you may be able to stand against the wiles of the devil. For we do not wrestle against flesh and blood, but against principalities, against powers, against the rulers of the darkness of this age, against spiritual hosts of wickedness in the heavenly places. Therefore take up the whole armor of God, that you may be able to withstand in the evil day, and having done all, to stand. Stand therefore, having girded your waist with truth, having put on the breastplate of righteousness, and having shod your feet with the preparation of the gospel of peace; above all, taking the shield of faith with which you will be able to quench all the fiery darts of the wicked one. And take the helmet of salvation, and the sword of the Spirit, which is the word of God; praying always with all prayer and supplication in the Spirit, being watchful to this end with all perseverance and supplication for all the saints—and for me, that utterance may be given to me, that I may open my mouth boldly to make known the mystery of the gospel, for which I am an ambassador in chains; that I may speak boldly, as I ought to speak. Ephesians 6:10-20 (NKJV)

I have been putting on the armor of God every time I wake up for many, many years. At one time I put it on out of order, but I learned God has reason why they are in that order. Now I put the armor on the way God has it in His Word, the Bible. I put it on the moment I am fully awake each time I wake up, even if only from a nap in the afternoon. It has made a difference in my life, a big, big difference. The best way to accomplish this process of putting on the armor of God is to memorize it.

Abba, gird my loins with the belt of truth: truth coming in, truth staying in and truth going out all at the same time. *Webster's Encyclopedia Dictionary of the English Language* defines gird as to bind with a girdle or flexible band; to encircle; to equip; to prepare, as, to gird oneself for battle. Gird my loins with the belt of truth: Not only are we to know God's truth, we are to obey God's truth. We are to be truthful and we are to share God's truth with others.

Place on my chest the breastplate of righteousness, the only thing that makes me righteous is Jesus' righteousness imputed to me. The only thing that makes me right with You, Abba, is Jesus.

Shod my feet with the thick boots of the gospel of peace, with a peace that passes all understanding in our hearts and minds. When I was very small, I would put my feet into my Daddy's work boots. They were so heavy I could not walk in them; I just stood in them. God's thick boots of the gospel of peace are big. They fit God's feet, but you can walk in His boots, He made it so you could.

Encompass me with the shield of faith, Your faith Jesus. There was a time I did not feel protected with this shield of faith. It was when I was in bed, and my back was vulnerable. Then I learned to ask God to encompass me, to encircle me with His shield of faith. That made the difference.

Place on my head the helmet of salvation, which is a day by day by day continuing process. Satan's playground is in our minds, so be sure you get this part of the armor on.

And place in my hands the Sword of the Spirit the Word of God. It is next to impossible to get God's Word in you unless you pick it up and read it. So get God's Word in your hands daily. Please place in my hands, into my heart, into my mind, will, emotions, body, soul, spirit and down into the very bone marrow of my soul Your sword of the Holy Spirit—the Word of God. I praise You and I thank You. Help me learn Your Word the Bible by heart. For I ask in Jesus' Name and to His glory, Amen.

Bro. Ted asked me to say the Armor of God during one of our church services. I had memorized it out of order and I became confused when he tried to help me say it, and I could not. Right after that I memorized it in the right order as it is in the Bible.

(9)

It Was Just a Feeling

I came to a time in my life when I thought it would be better if I were dead. I remember a feeling; it was always a feeling that triggered my suicide attempts. It was a feeling of lostness, beyond help, beyond being forgiven, beyond hope, darkness, aloneness, and despair. I left no note. I did not tell anyone. I just hurt inside and did not know how to stop the hurting. I just wanted the world to stop and let me off. I did not want to live anymore. Not like that, not anymore. There was no wound, nothing physically wrong with me. I just hurt on the inside and nothing helped. So one night I took a few bottles of pills at the house and drove my car out to the pasture we own. I went into the trailer house that was used for storage out there and lay down to die. Suicide is not the answer.

You shall not murder. Exodus 20:13 (NKJV)

I was saved, but still that overwhelming feeling of being lost was there. Feelings are temporal; they change all the time. I go up and down. But sometimes when I go down, it is a downward spiral. I do not talk to anyone, and I do not listen to anyone. I close the whole world out. I just wanted to go to sleep and never wake up ever again.

But God!

I did not die. That still was not good news to me. I did not want to live, not that way. My decision was to create a permanent solution to a temporary problem.

(10)

Momma's Account of the Story

*M*omma and Daddy raised honey bees, and we had gone to Bee Club in town. Afterwards we went to the grocery store. We bought corned beef and some tapioca pudding. About 9:00 or 10:00 o'clock we were home. Momma was tired, and I told her I was going to make tapioca pudding. She did not like the pudding, so she went on to bed. Daddy and I ate the pudding and talked for about an hour or so. Then he went to bed.

They awoke the next morning, and Daddy got ready to go to work about 6:00 o'clock. He came back in and said, "Carol's car is not here. Is she supposed to be going somewhere?" We were supposed to be having a prayer group, so Momma said she would give me about an hour. Daddy went on to work south of where we live. Momma checked my medications—it all seemed to be there. About 7:00 o'clock Momma still had not heard from me, so she called my in-laws and drove around—out to the pig patch and to the pasture outside of town, but she did not see my car. She decided she needed to stay by the phone in case something had happened to me. She called several people checking to see if they had seen me, nobody had. My Uncle Eddie (Momma's brother) went out to the pasture late that afternoon; he went in the west side gate. He came back out just as Daddy came back from work.

Daddy stopped to see what was going on. My uncle asked if they had found Carol yet. Daddy said, "No, not when he had called home." My uncle said, "I think I saw her car on the side road at the south gate." So they went to the south gate and went up to the trailer house. That is where they found me.

Uncle Eddie went to the house and got Momma. She grabbed a few clothes, knowing she would probably be spending the night with me. Daddy took me straight to the hospital, where they pumped my stomach. It had been a very cold night, and I did not have on a coat, which slowed down my metabolism. Dr. Greer said I would not have lasted another 30 minutes. He said there was to be no one but Momma or Daddy in the room with me. Within days they moved me to another hospital. That is when I was evaluated, and my psychiatrist started the electric shock treatments—14 of them. That is Momma's story of how it happened.

(11)

Sex Outside of Marriage is Sin

I came out of the hospital, but was later put back in and had from four to six more electric shock treatments. It triggered a manic phase. I came out of the hospital this time with a boy friend. I was having sex with him, and I was not married to him. I loved him and he loved me. He had a drinking problem, and he died in a car wreck due to drinking and driving. I thought it was my fault. I blamed me even if no one else did. It was a long time before I felt alive again. I praise God for Daniel. I thank God for my time with him, but my relationship with him was sin. It does not matter how I felt; I cannot get around the sin issue.

Do you not know that your bodies are members of Christ? Shall I then take the members of Christ and make them members of a harlot? Certainly not! Or do you not know that he who is joined to a harlot is one body with her? For "the two," He says, "shall become one flesh." But he who is joined to the LORD is one spirit with Him. Flee sexual immorality. Every sin that a man does is outside the body, but he who commits sexual immorality sins against his own body. Or do you not know that your body is the temple of the Holy Spirit who is in you, whom you have from God, and you are not your own? For you were bought at a price; therefore glorify God in your body and in your spirit, which are God's. 1 Corinthians 6:15-20 (NKJV)

Abba Father, forgive me for having sex outside of marriage. Forgive me, cleanse me, heal me, and restore me to a right spirit and relationship with You, LORD Jesus. I want first love back again with You. I want to love You again, please forgive me. Blot out this sin in my life right now. I confess my sin to You LORD.

Abba, help me love Jesus the way He deserves to be loved. Teach me agape love. I want to love Him more. I want to be a woman after God's own heart. Please help me. Holy Spirit fill me with Your love. Restore unto me the joy of Thy salvation. I thank You and I praise You, because You are worthy of praise. I do not know why some live and some die. I thank You for Your mercy and love and that I am alive. I thank You for Daniel and that my boyfriend was a Christian and that he is in heaven with You and alcohol has no control over him now. Thank You for healing me. I give You all the honor, credit and glory. In Jesus Name, Amen.

(12)

Suicide is Not an Answer

I hope you noticed the verses from the Bible I have written by the events in my life. They are there as reminders to me...Remember I had read the Ten Commandments in my Bible as a child and at the time I did not think I was guilty of any of them. God showed me I was guilty. God showed me I needed Him. God delivered me from pornography, sex outside of marriage, drinking, lying and stealing.

Jen, my daughter, came for a visit one summer and started living with us again. I would like to say, once I was saved that I never left the LORD, but I cannot. While Jen, Jay and I were living in our apartment, they would go to church, but I would stay home on Sundays. I was like that for months and months. I was so tired I could not get up out of bed.

Remember the Sabbath and keep it holy. Exodus 20:8 A (NKJV)

I did start going to church again. But I did not feel anything, I did not feel love, and I sure did not feel joy.

I beseech (that means urge) *you therefore, brethren, by the mercies of God, that you present your bodies a living sacrifice, holy, acceptable to God, which is your reasonable service.* Romans 12:1 (NKJV)

Another time I could not do it. I planned it. I found a syringe at Goo Goo's house. I had learned that if you get air in your veins, it could kill you. I checked out a book from the library to learn about blood vessels and veins. I spent one whole night trying to decide to try. My counselor came the next morning on a house visit. When I would not talk to her, she knew something was wrong. The police picked me up and took me to the State Hospital.

Another time I took pills again. All night long my heart raced and felt as if it was going to beat right out of my chest. Morning came, and I was still alive. So I grabbed another bottle of pills and took all of them, too. Those pills only made me throw up. Momma came home from work at noon, and I told her I needed to go to the hospital. They made me drink liquid charcoal. The doctor on call at the hospital emergency room said my heart was beating like a rabbit's. I went home the next day and life went on as if nothing had happened.

When did I get saved? I do not know. Maybe God saved a little girl who was so slow of thought but reached out to Him anyway. Maybe God worked with me and taught me until I was able to say those words out loud—"I believe in Jesus." God does not give me all the answers. I praise God—He knows the answers. He understands.

I wrote this to try to pinpoint exactly when I was saved and even after I finished I still did not know when I was saved. So I asked God and He told me I was saved when I knelt down on my knees at the trailer house that day in east Texas. He continues to save me daily. When did you get saved?

Forgiveness—past, present and future

Justification—just as if I had never sinned

Sanctification—an ongoing process

Glorification—till people see Jesus in me

Because God wants a living sacrifice, I do not try to take my life anymore. It just is not an option for me anymore.

Abba, forgive me for picking up that first pornography magazine that led to others and forgive me for having sex outside of marriage. Forgive me for drinking too much. Forgive me for stealing over and over and over again. Forgive me for lying. Thank You for deliverance in these areas.

I need You now, God. I need to see Your hand in all of this. I do not understand. If I do not take my medicine, I get sick. I do not function. I tried to kill myself; over and over I have tried it. Depression is dark and dry and lonely. Manic is destructive. Is this a test? If it is, I am failing it. I need You, God. I need You. Forgive me, I do not know what the answer is because I do not know what the question is. Do I abuse drugs? I have before. I have taken too many drugs at different times trying to kill myself. I am sorry. Forgive me. You want a living sacrifice not a dead one.

Abba Father, thank You that I am alive. I praise You, God. God has a purpose and a plan for good and not for evil and a future and a promise of hope. I praise You God that I am alive. You are the only reason that I am, but come quickly LORD Jesus, come quickly. Thank You for healing me over and over again. Thank You for walking me to the other side of depression and back down from manic over and over again. Abba Father, thank You and I praise You that I never seemed to fit in anywhere in this world until I came to You, Jesus. And You made it all right. You complete me. In Jesus Name, the Most Precious Name I know, Amen.

(13)

Medication

ॐ

I depend on pills. I take a lot. I take a vitamin, calcium, high blood pressure medicine. I am diabetic, but it is diet controlled. I take a medicine for cholesterol and a medicine because I get car sick, air sick when I fly, and sea sick when I am on the ocean. I take an allergy medicine because I am allergic to so many things: ragweed, mountain cedar, wasp, horses, band aids and tapes and now the doctor says I am allergic to the sun and gravel.

I started taking different medicines at first for major depression and then many years later for manic depression also called bipolar. Not until today did I understand how much I was dependent on it. I have to gradually come off my medicine for bipolar. I do not want to feel like this. And right now I am not even completely off it yet. I am still able to sleep at night because I am still taking two medicines to help me sleep, but Tuesday I have to stop taking one of those. I am not looking forward to it. I cannot handle it now. I could not handle it yesterday.

These have been hard days, days without peace, days of physically hurting, days of no rest. I sleep through the night because of the Zyprexa till 2:30 or 4:00 or 6:00 and then I am up. I cannot seem to pray. So I went back to my prayers I had written down. And it was sweet. And it was time with

You, LORD, but I cannot relax! I am coming off Tegretal which I have been on for five years. At the same time I am going on Celexa an anti-depressant. So, Abba how much of this is withdrawal and how much is the burden of unconfessed and undealt with sin in my life? All I know is I need more than Your help. I need You to live in me. I want to be in the very throne room of heaven with You, and I need Jesus to live in my body. I need You to feel what this feels like because I cannot seem to explain it to You. Show up and be in me. LORD Jesus, show up and be big.

August Monday AM 8-18-08

Abba, this morning the tremors started. I was shaking uncontrollably. I told You I cannot take this anymore, just like I told You yesterday, Sunday. I cannot take this anymore. I asked You, Abba and Jesus and Your Holy Spirit, the complete Trinity, to invade my body. Come and make Your home in me. Yesterday all three of You lived in me, and today I know You all are in me, because You say if we ask believing that You will answer our prayers. You are all in me. The tremors stopped. As I fixed breakfast this morning, I asked You, God, if You can invade my body like that, can You invade my—sub conscious, unconscious, conscious mind, my will, emotions, body, soul, spirit and heart? And You did! I do not want to get complacent. I do not want to get slack. When things get better, I do not want to forget I need You in me just as much as I need You now. I do not want to forget what those tremors felt like. Some people today are trying to stop taking drugs, or alcohol, and they are having the tremors—I pray for them, too. I pray someone will tell them they need You, God and Jesus and the Holy Spirit in their lives. I pray for victory in Jesus. I pray for victory for them too. Please save people today all over the world. We have today with no promise of tomorrow. Help me tell someone today that You God the Trinity are the answer to any problem in our lives. Help me keep on telling it to as many people as will listen. In Jesus Name, Amen.

I am dependent on the medicine I take, but I depend on God for my healing. He walks me through depression or manic back to a sound mind and a calm spirit. I have to keep taking my medicine but I also have to keep telling my doctors what that medicine is doing so it can be monitored and regulated according to how I am doing on it. That means I see my doctors regularly too and do what they say. If I do not, I could end up in the state hospital or dead.

It is no sin to feel helpless. It is right where God wants you, so you will turn to Him so He can help you. The shortest prayer there is: "Help, Jesus!" You do not have to explain to God how He needs to help you. Just trust Him that He knows the best way to handle it. But He wants to hear your conversation with Him about it in prayer. Remember, prayer is talking to God and listening to God. And if you forget His instructions just become still and quiet and silently in your heart ask Him to repeat Himself and He will. He does not get mad because we forgot. But He does not like it when we have been told and we understand what He says to do and we do not do it.

I could stay in bed all day, but that would not be good, so I try to stay busy and keep my mind occupied with the right things. I also have to rest too, so it cannot be all of one or the other, but both, working and resting. Sometimes I did not even care to get out of bed to eat much less take my medicine, but I had to take my medicine. I made a pinky promise with my pastor at the time, when I was in the state hospital that I would eat and it has stuck.

There is something wrong, and I do not know how to fix it. Bro. Randy says if it is not broken do not fix it. Well I am broken, but that is what I pray for daily—"Break me, bend me, tear me, and crush me." I want to be broken bread and poured out wine for You, LORD.

The sacrifices of God are a broken spirit, A broken and a contrite heart—These, O God, You will not despise.
Psalm 51:17 (NKJV)

Abba, for so long I have second guessed what the medicine would do to me. How I was suppose to act. It cannot be acting any more. But I cannot go by my feelings anymore either. What do I do? I do not know if I am up or down. It feels like pressure weighing on me. It hurts; physically hurts. I do not want to feel like this. Everyone says stay on the medicine, but with me, I get allergic to the medicines after a time. Thank You and I praise You—it has been five years since I have had to change my medicine or be in the state hospital. You do not want us to take the edge off life with drugs, not even prescription drugs. You want us to feel life. Pain—we would not know something is wrong usually without the pain to tell us.

Abba, a broken and contrite heart You will not turn away. Am I asking amiss? Do I need to stop asking to be broken? At the same time I ask to be broken I also ask You—"mend me and heal me."

They call depression a cloud, a shadow, but this one hurts. A shadow cannot touch you but this shadow does. I do not really remember when this shadow of depression started coming over me? How far back does it go? I remember times as a child on the school playground when I did not play—I just stood by the wall. I remember times in Jr. High as I first started having to change classes from teacher to teacher and room to room that I did not do that well. I spent many mornings in the bathroom sick at my stomach. I remember when I left the town I grew up in after I got married—I just stayed in bed or on the couch trying to sleep the pain away. Daily I would watch *MASH, Little House on the Prairie* and *The Waltons* reruns on TV, and I would cry through most of it. But I could not put a name to it. After Jay was born, I went into a deep depression, post partum depression. It happened in an instant. It just came over me. Was it sin? Is that the root cause? That is what I am asking You, LORD, is my depression a sin against You? Forgive me. It is not anyone else's fault. Is it my fault? Am I doing something wrong? Is this a thorn in the flesh? I pray for a spirit of humility. God keep me humble and childlike, yet mature spiritually. In Jesus Name, Amen.

(14)

A Way of Life

*G*luttony is a hard sin, because it is not like alcohol or drugs. We have to eat. We cannot just put it down and never eat another bite. God, You have taught me certain things that help. I went through the *Weighdown* program by Gwen Shamblin twice. It cost a lot of money, but it is well worth it for her advice, input, and the scripture to back it up. Through the Weighdown Workshop:

> I learned what true hunger feels like to me and it is different with different people.
> I learned the difference between head hunger and real hunger.
> I learned that sometimes I ate because — just because. I ate because I did not feel good, and I was trying to comfort myself with food or sometimes I was just bored or sometimes I would eat out of habit and it was just "time" to eat.
> I learned to eat out of a salad plate — not the huge dinner plate or even the middle size plate but the small salad size plate. I know it is psychological, but I put a lot on my salad plate. It looks full to me, and I know when I am finished I have had a meal.
> I learned to drink glasses of water — all through the day. It fills me up, and even if I am eating less food, it still satis-

fies me and I do not feel hungry until I hear my stomach growl. That is how I know I am hungry, but that is different for different people. Some feel a burning sensation in their stomach, and there are other ways to tell when you are hungry.

I eat dessert—dessert may only be a piece of fruit or a bunch of grapes, sometimes it is a mini candy bar or a small piece of cake with frosting on the top only and not on the sides or one cookie. I am borderline diabetic, and it is diet controlled and it is not with sugar free foods. I lost weight. I eat fresh fruits, and canned fruits in natural juice and dried fruit. I may only drink a quarter of a cup of juice at a meal. I get tired of the same foods over and over, so I go for variety. God gave us an abundance of different foods. I choose healthy foods. I eat a variety of fresh, raw and cooked vegetables. I go for color, the more color and the deeper the color the better. I go for texture, a variety of textures. I eat all kinds of meat: fish, poultry, beans and nuts. I eat bread, rice and pasta. I drink milk, juices, tea, coffee, herb teas, hot spiced tea, hot spiced apple cider. I eat what I crave, just in moderation. I learned if I overeat, the blood in my brain is diverted to my stomach and it makes me sleepy, if I do not overeat, I have more energy to do the things I want to do in life and I do not sleep all day.

I do not have to eat all the time at breakfast time, or lunch time or supper time. Sometimes I do eat at a meal time, but not always. I eat breakfast because I have to take my morning medicine with food.

It is no diet—it is a way of life I can live with and be satisfied with every day of my life.

I learned scriptures and what God has to say about food in the Bible.

God blesses my efforts.

I praise God and thank Him.

I thank God for Gwen Shamblin.

Abba, forgive me for placing so much value on a meal or snack that will be digested in a matter of hours. Thank You that food does not mean as much to me now as before. Thank You and I praise You for the weight I have lost. I pray to be a healthy weight, I do not want to be thin, but I do not want to weigh too much either. Thank You, God for the variety of food. Help me not to overeat. Thank You for Your forgiveness. Thank You for Your love. Help me not to seek the comfort of food anymore but to seek the comfort and peace the Holy Spirit gives. In Jesus Name, Amen.

(15)

The State Hospital

I have been baptized three times. I did not feel saved. Many were the times as I walked out the doors of the church—I was reminded I was not saved—and time was running out. I was put in the state hospital two more times. I thank God for the people who prayed for me. Prayer makes all the difference. God listens when you pray.

When I was in the state hospital for the first time, a post card from my neighbor and a prayer from my pastor made a difference. For weeks I had the sensation that I was being burned with a blazing inferno of fire on the inside of my body. I tried taking cold showers, it did not help. Cold baths did not help. My pastor at that time came to the hospital and we talked. I told him what was happening, and we prayed living water on me. I praise God the burning went away. A post card from my neighbor was of a waterfall, and it was something I could carry in the pocket of my sweater to remind me of God's living water and how God had answered our prayer. I took it out and looked at it any time I needed a reminder of what God had done in my life.

"He who believes in Me, as the Scripture has said, out of his heart will flow rivers of living water." John 7:38 (NKJV)

The next time I was in the State Hospital, I was bad. I did things I should not have. But my pastor Bro. Ricky and our music director, Bro. Jim would tell me week after week, Jesus said, "I will never leave you nor forsake you." That is what Jesus promises. He said it to me until I began to believe it was true. The Holy Spirit tells me now, "I will never leave you nor forsake you." He says it over and over again and then He says, "I will tell you that as many times as you need to hear it.

Do not hide Your face from me; Do not turn Your servant away in anger; You have been my help; Do not leave me nor forsake me, O God of my salvation. Psalm 27:9 (NKJV)

And the LORD, He is the One who goes before you. He will be with you, He will not leave you nor forsake you; do not fear nor be dismayed." Deuteronomy 31:8 (NKJV)

Let your conduct be without covetousness; be content with such things as you have. For He Himself has said, "I will never leave you nor forsake you." So we may boldly say: "The LORD is my helper; I will not fear. What can man do to me?" Hebrews 13:5-6 (NKJV)

I have been in the state hospital in north central Texas two different times for a total of four months. When I was in the state hospital for three months the devil lied to me, he told me one day that God had died. The next day he told me Jesus had died. Then the next day he told me the Holy Spirit had died. But God, God would not quit talking to me. When I would bow my head before I ate my meals, God talked, And when I woke up at four in the morning to take my bath, God would meet with me on my knees by my bed. He was not dead.

The last time I was in there the devil called me Marionette for weeks on end. I was a human puppet on his strings. There was a chasm below me. The strings kept me suspended in air in my mind. I would walk back and forth, to and fro. Finally one day the strings got so tangled that I could no longer take another step. In that moment I waited to see what would happen next. The strings that held me tight were cut. But God, instead of falling into the deep, dark abyss, I walked away free from the knots and tangles of the strings, free from the puppeteer. I did not fall, I walked away that day changed forever. God freed me from the devil's clutches, and he never tried it again. I praise God. I thank God.

The people who worked in the state hospital had keys to all the doors and I did not have a key to get out. I still have a fear of being locked in or locked out even to this day. I always check my keys to see if I have them, so I can get in or out as the case may be. Bro. Jim, our music minister, would come to visit me while I was in the state hospital during the time I was there for three months. I have learned over the years I am not alone anymore. Jesus is with me all the time. One of the names of Jesus is Immanuel. Immanuel means God with us. He really does never leave us nor forsake us. And He is closer than our very breath.

Bro. Jim and Bro. Ricky, my pastor at that time, would pray with me. I thank God for them, what they said, and for their prayers. I could not pray. I would get up early each morning and get on my knees before Holy God. But I could not put into words what was on my heart. I learned later in small group, which met at Momma and Daddy's house during 40 Days of Purpose by Rick Warren, from Bro. Jim that there are times the Holy Spirit intercedes for us with groaning which cannot be uttered. God met me there each morning I got on my knees in the hospital even if I could not put words into prayers.

I did get out of the state hospital after three months. It took longer because the doctor was trying to find the right medications for me, and I did not have electric shock treatments. I consider the Holy Spirit to be the best Counselor of all time. I needed a counselor 7 days a week — 24 hours a day — every minute of every hour—every second of every minute of the day, every day. I needed more than a doctor could give me.

You see the Holy Spirit knew my thoughts before I thought them. He knew me — what I was really like. He knew why I did the things I did—better than I knew myself. He knew the questions to ask me. And above all else—the Holy Spirit knew the answers. No counselor or doctor even comes close. I praise God for His Holy Spirit.

I would be dead if Jesus and God my Abba, Father and God the Holy Spirit had not loved me back to the living. I needed Their love and forgiveness, Their support, Their comfort, Their correction, Their friendship, Their healing and especially Their presence in my life.

I needed more than doctors and counselors could do for me. I would not talk to them or anyone else about my problems or what was happening in my life. One of the names for the Holy Spirit is Counselor. Dr. Jeff, a psychiatrist that is in my family, once told me a counselor is someone who sells you on an idea. The Holy Spirit is my Counselor, He sold me on Jesus. But I learned that though I could not talk to people about my problems, I could talk to my Abba, Father. Abba means God is a DADDY, my DADDY and He can be your DADDY too and He is available both day and night.

Behold, He who keeps Israel shall neither slumber nor sleep. Psalm 121:4 (NKJV)

God is who I had always longed for. He meets my inmost needs. I found Jesus to be my very Best Friend. He loves me. I can talk to Him about anything. Maybe you have a need in your life today. Jesus is the answer to any problem you may have to face. He is a good listener because He can do something about our problems if we just ask. God does not always answer me the way I think He will answer me. But God always forgives us of our sins when we ask Him. Trust Jesus, He is the answer to any problem you are going through right now, or in your past or even in your future. He can forgive you of anything except not asking for forgiveness in the first place. God can use even the bad things that happen to us in our lives and bring good out of them when we bring them to Him.

For I know the plans I have for you, says the LORD. They are plans for good and not for evil, to give you a future and a hope. Jeremiah 29:11 (TLB)

That is my life verse.

*****

David Livingston said about God's Word:

"It is the word of a Gentleman of the most sacred and strictest honor, and there's an end to it!"

I have that written in the front of my Bible. Jesus will not break down the door to your heart, but He knocks and patiently waits for you to open that door. If you still cannot do that today, and if you have become convinced that God does not exist, will you please pray a simple prayer to whom you believe to be a nonexistent God.

God, if you are real, help me to believe. In Jesus Name, Amen.

Jesus is a Gentleman; He will not barge in on your life. You have to ask Him in.

Abba, thank You for freedom. Thank You that You would not let me go. I do not like the devil, he tricks me, lies to me and takes advantage of me. Thank You God that You are nothing like the devil. You tell me the truth, You guide my every step. You do the impossible, the improbable and always the right thing to do. You are alive forever. You saved me and You protect me. Thank You that You are always here with me by Your Holy Spirit. Thank You God that You and Jesus are in Heaven and that Jesus prays for me and for all Christians. Thank You

Jesus that You pray for the lost to be saved. LORD of the harvest send forth labors into Your harvest fields. Save the lost, heal the sick and raise the dead. Speak softly, lovingly to comfort the grieving. Thank You for joy not interrelated with what happens in my life. I love You Abba, I love You Jesus and I love You Holy Spirit. I pray for revival. I pray for Spiritual Awakening. Not just for me but for everyone in the whole world. Blow the fires of revival until the lost would be saved and the saved would tell the lost about Jesus who saved them. Jesus, You are not coming back until we do. Forgive me, I do not talk to people. I want to be bold. I want to be brave. I want to be courageous. I think everyone needs You, Jesus. Help me open my mouth and speak to the glory of God. Thank You for saving me from that serpent the devil and telling me that the devil was the one telling the lies. Thank You, forever thank You. I worship You and I praise You forever and ever more. I ask in the Name above all names, Jesus. Amen.

(16)

Do you Have Anything to Give to Jesus?

❧

One Sunday morning Bro. Ricky preached about a little boy who did not have anything to give to Jesus. The little boy placed the offering plate down on the ground and got in it. The little boy gave himself to Jesus. Ever since that day I lay down, each morning now, my face on the floor and prayerfully put me in God's offering plate. That is how I start my day. God honors that decision every day. I also put on the armor of God, piece by piece, each morning. It does not weigh anything and you cannot see it but you sure can tell when it is on. It is my Heavenly Father's so it is big enough to protect me.

Jesus taught me another thing; being saved is not a feeling. Feelings change, they are temporal—that means temporary. Feelings change all the time. Trusting Jesus to save you is a fact. Jesus saves completely; you can count on it all the time, no matter how you feel that particular day.

while we look not at the things which are seen, but at the things which are not seen; for the things which are seen are temporal, but the things which are not seen are eternal. 2 Corinthians 4:18 (NASB)

Do I make all the right decisions—no—I still sin. But when I confess them to God and ask for forgiveness, He forgives. God has taught me to be very specific when I confess my sin to Him. He knows all about it anyway. But I need to know my sin, so I can forsake it—that means to turn away from my sin and not do it anymore, that is called repentance. God deals with one sin at a time in my life because that is all I can deal with at a time.

I went to Glorietta to the Baptist Encampment a few years ago with a group of divorced single men and women. It is a wonderful place to go and get closer to God. I went to the early morning devotional time out among the trees. I went to the prayer garden and just sat and prayed, walked with God and talked to Him. I learned something in one of the sessions on which I still depend:

Open your hand that you do not use for writing. Use a Sharpie and draw a stick figure in the palm of your hand and close that hand you drew on. If you belong to Christ, Jesus wraps His hands around you. Then God the Father wraps both His hands around Jesus' hands (close your other hand around the one on which you just drew the stick figure). You cannot see Him, but the Holy Spirit wraps His hands around Jesus' and God the Father's hands. Nothing can ever snatch you out of His and Their hands. Nothing! Nothing! Nothing!

Abba, I praise You for truth upon truth. I have had to draw that stick figure in my hand and do this as a reminder of You holding me in Your hands. When the Sharpie washes off, I put it right back on again and again until the object lesson speaks tons of faith to my soul. Thank You that even when I cannot hold on to You, You continue to hold me in Your hands. I cannot fall out of Your hands. Thank You for the opportunity to go to Glorietta, New Mexico. I learned much, I learned much! I praise You LORD. Thank You. In Jesus Name, Amen.

(17)

Tears are Very Healing

"*C*ry me a handful of tears". Someone said that to me a lot when I was a child. I would stop crying and sometimes I would laugh at him. I have cried a lot of tears in my lifetime of 53 years. God holds every tear drop; mine and yours if you are reading this. God has big hands and He catches every tear drop. But after I had cried so much one day years ago, I asked God if I could just quit crying. And He answered my prayer. I quit crying.

Abba, it hurts worse when we cannot cry tears. Please make null and void my prayer to You for me to quit crying tears. Please help me cry again and know that You catch every tear drop. Thank You and I praise You. Forgive me for asking You to stop my tears. It hurts too much not to cry real tears. Please help me not to be ashamed of crying. Help me know it is safe to cry. That it is not only okay, but also very, very much a part of the healing process. Soften my heart with the tears. Help us taste the saltiness of our tears. You created us that way, laughter and tears, and sometimes we can laugh and cry in the very same moment, like when we watch the cemetery scene, in the movie, *Steel Magnolias*. I pray for the tears, but I pray to laugh again with the joy of the LORD not contingent upon what happens in my life. No matter what this day brings, I pray for a peace that You are in control and so everything is okay. Help me not to go on feelings. Feelings are temporal. That means they are changing all the time. So as Beth Moore puts it "I choose joy. It has been appropriated to me, and I choose joy."

Why, Abba Daddy, did I not know to ask You to forgive me of my sin and that in Jesus Name we can ask to be forgiven and You forgive? Why? Why did it take me so long to come to You? Why? In Jesus Name, Amen.

(18)

Financial Freedom

*I*n February 2008 of this year I started another journey with God. I went to a Crown Financial Bible study. The group was comprised of Kristi, Amy, Crystal, Lorraine, and me. There were five of us. I learned so much more than just about money. I learned scripture memorization and accountability to other people. I learned to listen to others viewpoint. I learned to trust others advice. I learned I do not have to spend all my money. I can give 10% to God. I can save some, spend some and invest some. I can invest in God's kingdom, by sending it on ahead of me into Heaven by investing my time, talents, and treasure into God's capable hands and His kingdom. When people get saved, they go to heaven. I want as many people to get saved as can be before Jesus comes back. I want Satan to be so very disappointed at how few there are left behind when the rapture does happen. If I want that, then just think about how much more God wants that. God is not sending Jesus back until the last person who can be saved will be saved before the rapture. Do you want Jesus to come back? We can give to those who are telling others about Jesus. But it is going to take every one of us telling people whom we come into daily contact, about Jesus instead of talking about the weather, gossiping or chit chatting. We have today with no promise of tomorrow. Invest in the kingdom of God; tell someone what you know about Jesus, and what He has done in your life. Today! I do not have a lot of money but the Crown financial ministries taught me it is not about the thousand dollars I do not have, it is all about the ten dollars that I do have.

I was not seeking God's guidance about handling my finances, and I could not keep enough money in the bank. This sin distanced me from God. He let me spend the money my way, but I had leanness in my soul. I did not have a relationship with God. We cannot love both God and money. What I got I could not keep. We built a new house—we did not even get to live in it a year before we had to sell it. I did not get to be with my daughter while she was in elementary school. When I started giving to the LORD, God started giving back to me. It was not always with money but with blessings money could not buy. God blessed me with a son and a daughter to love. God blessed me abundantly with homes in which to stay: Nanny and Pa, Momma and Daddy, Uncle Kyle and Aunt Wanda, the lake house, Aunt Sue and Uncle Kenneth and sometimes with Babe.

Abba, forgive me. For so long, I thought if I earned the money, then it was my money. Now I see that it is all Yours— even the 90% leftover from the tithe to You, is all Yours, God. Help me tithe and spend a little and save a little. Steady plodding. It is no quick fix. It is a journey with You, teach me obedience to You and help me make wise choices in where Your money is to go. Help me be a hilarious giver. Help us get back together to start meeting and sharing what You have been doing since the last time we went through the Crown Financial Ministries Seminar. Help us divide up into groups. I pray and ask that others will be open and want to go through the seminar and learn what the Bible has to say to us about money and how we are to invest our time, talent, and treasure in Your kingdom.

Abba, thank You, I do not own a house, but You have blessed me with homes in which to stay when needed. Thank You for SSI-SSDI. Thank You and I praise You for Ms.

Susanne and John at the Social Security office. Thank You that after Jen and Jay left for a time, they came back. Thank You for their friendship and their love. Thank You for the white car Bro. Randy let me drive for a while. Thank You for the money You provide to live on and some to give back to You at church. Thank You for Amy, Crystal, Kristi, and Lorraine and the Crown financial teaching we have been learning. It has made a huge difference knowing You are in control of everything, even Your money. It takes the pressure off by spending, saving and giving God's way. In Jesus Name, Amen.

(19)

Missing God's Best

A lot of time I react before I get clear instruction from God. I tend to hear one instruction and try to do it when if I had waited and kept listening to God it would have helped. I tend to react and do something right then instead of waiting on God. I miss God's best. I miss the journey with Him. I short change God. I do not get the big picture, only a corner piece, or maybe a piece out of the center of the puzzle called life. Life happens fast. If you are not ready for it; it can run over you.

I did not care enough to ask how others were doing or to take the time and concern enough to listen to what they said. There was sin of indifference in my prayer life, too. If I do not know them personally, I tended not to pray for them. I need God's love, love enough to care, love enough to give away. I miss opportunities to witness and love. I miss getting to know people. If I do not reach out to others, I am in my own little world and I do not let anyone else in. People are important to God.

But when the kindness and love of God our Savior toward man appeared, not by works of righteousness which we have done, but according to His mercy He saved us, through the washing of regeneration and renewing of the Holy Spirit, whom He poured out on us abundantly through Jesus Christ our Savior, that having been justified by His grace we should become heirs according to the hope of eternal life. Titus 3:4-7 (NKJV)

Abba, forgive me; so many times I get the cart before the horse. You can tell me one thing, and I go off trying to do it when if I had just stayed still and silent longer You might have given me more instructions. I made lots of trips to town. If I had written my list down, I could have gotten it all done in one trip. You have taught me to write "Jesus" in a box in the center of my list. I write all around Your Name what I have to do that day and therefore I keep my focus on You, Jesus, where it belongs. Abba, forgive me—there is no telling how much gas I have wasted. I like this way better, Jesus is my reason for living. You are responsible for my still being alive and I praise You and thank You. Thank You for all who have prayed for me to get well. God bless their lives. Thank You for Your prayers for me, Abba and Jesus and Your Holy Spirit. Thank You for prayer partners, especially Carolyn, Bro. Randy and Pam. Thank You for Dr. Snowden, Dr. Wieck, Dr. Greer and Dr. Tom. Thank You for prayer and answered prayer. Thank You that sometimes You answer "no" and that is the best answer You can give at the time. Thank You that sometimes Your answer will not come until we get to heaven. Abba, help, Abba, forgive me.

Abba, indifference to me means I did not really care about other people. People are important to You. We cost You Your Son Jesus' life. He was able to pick His life back up again; thank You, God; that He was able to pick His life back up again. It is finished. Jesus' work on the cross is finished, and He will not ever have to die to pay that price again. The sacrifice, the lamb, was brought over and over again in the Old Testament of the Bible, but payment was in full when the Lamb, Jesus Christ, was slain for our sins once for all. Abba, forgive me. Help me care, really care, about other people. I pray to love people with Your love. I pray for mercy and peace. I pray for Your compassion. I pray that I will have a tender heart towards other people. Jesus saved us, not because of righteous things we had done, but because of His mercy, grace and love. Thank You God for Your mercy. Thank You for Your grace. Thank You for Your love. Help me not to be afraid of people. Help me have a healthy fear of You, God. Help me care about people I may never see face to face. People are important to You; let them be important to me, too. Give me the love with which to love them, even for those who will never love me in return. In Jesus Name, Amen.

(20)

Bible Study

If you ever get a chance to go hear Beth Moore speak, go! If you ever have a chance to do a Bible study by Beth Moore, do it! Do not worry if you do not get all your homework done. That has happened to all of us at some time or other, but be there for every session to fellowship and pray together and worship with the other ladies or men in the Bible study. Go every time to see the video of Beth's teaching. She is an excellent teacher, and although I have never talked face to face with her, she is my mentor, and I consider her one of my closest friends. I have done ten Bible studies under her leadership, and I have never regretted one of them. Sometimes I have to finish my homework after we are through with the Bible study, but I try to always go even if I did not get through with a lesson. Beth teaches deep truths, and you have to work and be diligent to do the homework but it is well worth the effort involved. She has us turn the pages in our Bible. She says that it is her favorite sound. I think God smiles on us as we turn the pages in our Bibles and dig deeper into His Word than we do at other times when we aren't in the Bible study. I teach the three year olds during Sunday school, but I still need to be taught God's Word, and Beth does it so well. She does a lot of the work for us. She looks up the Greek and Hebrew words and tells us what they mean. She makes us laugh and cry. She shares, cares, and loves our LORD and us.

Abba, thank You and I praise You for Beth Moore. Thank You, God, for Keith, her husband. He prays for her and with her and for us. Thank You God for my sister in Christ, Beth, what a blessed gift You have given us by her friendship and teaching that comes across even on a video, and as we dig into God's Word, the Bible. God, I pray my prayers for her and even more because she has different needs than I do. Love her by meeting needs in her life only You and Beth know about. Help her family, friends, loved ones, associates, and even her enemies to come to You. I pray a special prayer that her Jewish friends will become completed Jews; please save them. Help her to know she is loved by You and by us. And according to Your will LORD, if it is okay, could Michael come back to Keith and Beth when he reaches 18 and is all grown up? But not my will but Yours be done. Thank You for all the teachers who have taught the Bible studies, Trish, Cindy and Carma. In Jesus Name, Amen.

(21)

Getting to Know You

*A*bba, where do I go from here? What is next? This is
to Your glory. That is what You have spoken over me;
I give You credit where credit is due. This is Your book. What
do we talk about next? I praise You and thank You that I am
manic. But do not let the manic get in the way of Your story.
Less of me and more of You, and I do not want to box You in. I
give You permission; we can talk about anything You want me
to talk about. You taught me last Saturday that I am forgiven—
past, present and future sins. That knowledge has taken the
burden away. It has freed me. I will talk to You about any area
of my life.

God, I judged people by what I saw on the outside instead
of what was on the inside of them. You have been working
on this sin through the years in me. How? You have placed
people who are different from me in my path. James and Suki,
J J and Tanya, Toledo and Mr. Geters, and the people at the
black church when we went there as a choir to sing, that is
where You first introduced me to James and Suki—James
sang that night and I sat next to them. They have become
very good friends. There was the lady who cooked a meal
for us when I went with my friends over to her house. I have
learned to love Tony Evans and his wife through their devo-
tionals they share with me and right now we are doing a Bible

study that his daughter Priscilla Shirer wrote part of. I have met Australians; I have met people from Okinawa. I have met people from Boston, and St. Louis. I have had Kamry and Selena in my Sunday school class. Thank You that I got to love them. I have met Meredith, Mark, Doug, and Katy. They have captured my heart.

Abba, You have placed Sandra, in my life and all the elderly people at the rest home and the home bound. They are a rich treasure in my heart and life. My grandparents are all with You in heaven, but You have blessed me with the privilege of getting to know these dear elderly brothers and sisters in Christ over the years. My life would be so empty without them. I praise You and thank You for my life is rich in these people and there is nothing wrong with any of them. There is everything very right about each and every one of them. Thank You for Bro. Randy and Pam, Bro. Jim and Sandra, Bro. Jimmy and Cindy. Thank You for all my dear friends; they make me want to try harder. Thank You.

Abba, I want to be color blind. I want to not even notice what color a person's skin is. I pray to not notice if someone is different from me—physically, mentally or spiritually. I am not "normal"; help me not to judge any other person. I am not the standard, God, You are. Help me measure up to You, Abba, Father. Help me not to judge! Forgive me. You did it right, Jesus, You never sinned. You paid the sin penalty for our sins when You died on the cross. Therefore it is Your righteousness imputed to us. I thank You and I praise You for Your forgiveness, Your mercy, Your grace, Your peace and Your love. I love You back because You first loved me. Perfect love casts out fear. Abba, help me see what is right about other people and that there is nothing "wrong" with any of them at all. I ask in the Blessed Name of my Jesus, Amen.

There is no fear in love; but perfect love casts out fear, because fear involves torment. But he who has fears has not been made perfect in love. 1 John 4:18-19 (NKJV)

I have missed out on meeting, getting to know and loving some really neat people because I judged them by their looks. If something is different about them that is what makes them special and unique and they usually have a lot more love to love me back than other people. When I did not judge them and overcame my prejudice I found out they are great people to know. They are loving people and my life would be so empty without them.

(22)

There is a Wedding to Attend

May of 2008

I learned this year that in the Jewish culture when someone is engaged to be married it is as if they are already married and the groom is already responsible for His bride to be. It is up to Him to make all the arrangements for the wedding including what the bride is to wear.

So I started asking God, my Abba Father, to teach me to dance so I would know how to at the marriage supper when God tells Jesus to go and get His bride, the church, which includes me and He takes His bride, the church, to heaven.

So I would slip into the bathroom at night when, either I would ask God to teach me to dance or God would ask me to dance with Him.

May 23rd through 25th of 2008 I went to a family reunion at the lake. I told my cousin, Jana, what I had been doing. That is when I learned about Steven Curtis Chapman's daughter's accident and death. That is when I learned about his "Cinderella" song. I went to Mardel's Christian Book Store and bought the "This Moment" CD. I have been praying for Steven and his family. I wanted to hear the "Cinderella" song, but all of the songs have ministered to me during this time in my life.

One night while I was dancing with God to the "Cinderella" song, I asked God, what does the Prince of Peace, Jesus, not know? I knew Jesus knows everything. But Abba, Father told me Jesus does not know the time, hour or moment when Abba, Father will turn to Him at the midnight hour and say to Him, "Jesus, go and get Your Bride." I say midnight because it will be the last hour that ushers out the church age. Nanny says it will be midnight somewhere on earth when Jesus comes back. It does not mean that the rapture necessarily will happen at midnight here where we are but that when the rapture happens it will be an ending of Christ's church age here on earth. "The clock will strike 'midnight' and she, the Bride of Christ, His church will be gone as we know it. It is called the rapture. Jesus will then start working with the Jews again.

In the mean time Jesus is interceding for us. He is praying for us, lifting us up before the Father on our behalf. Know that Jesus is praying for you until the clock strikes "midnight" and He comes back for us. Jesus is praying, and so am I.

There is a wedding feast to attend. Are we inviting anyone to be there? We do that by inviting people to get to know our Savior Jesus Christ in a close, personal, loving and intimate relationship. The wedding is a fact! Are we sending out the invitations?

(23)

Beginning Another Journey

I am manic depressive also called bipolar disorder. For about six months now I have been having trouble. I talked to the people who were at prayer meeting during spring break of 2008 and told them I was having trouble. They called me to the front and prayed and laid hands on me. Then Bro. Randy and I talked after prayer meeting was over. Bro. Randy told me I was to rest and eat for an indefinite time. He arranged for me to be off from work where I volenteer. He arranged for people to take my place during Wednesday night fellowship suppers, where I cook for the church.

I went home and rested and ate and rested and ate and rested and ate. Two weeks later I started cooking at the church again. Bro. Randy told me I could drive a car he had. I learned that God not only owns all the cattle on a 1,000 hills, He also owns all the cars. I praise God.

For every beast of the forest is Mine, And the cattle on a thousand hills. Psalm 50:10 (NKJV)

Do you not know that your bodies are members of Christ? Shall I then take the members of Christ and make them members of a harlot? Certainly not! Or do you not know that he who is joined to a harlot is one body with her? For "the two," He says, "shall become one flesh." But he who is joined to the Lord is one spirit with Him. Flee sexual immorality. Every sin that a man does is outside the body, but he who commits sexual immorality sins against his own body. Or do you not know that your body is the temple of the Holy Spirit who is in you, whom you have from God, and you are not your own? For you were bought at a price; therefore glorify God in your body and in your spirit, which are God's. 1 Corinthians 6:15-20 (NKJV)

Abba, You own all the cars too, and You are letting me drive one. I praise You. I thank You. Thank You for Bro. Bill and the van he let me drive. Thank You for Bro. Randy and the little white car he is letting me drive.

Abba, I do not know if I have done right or wrong. I met with Bro. Randy and Pam and I talked about why I needed accountability partners. I talked to them about my background of having sex with men in the general hospital and the state hospital. And now I am attracted to someone. I need Your help. I need Your guidance. I need You to tell me no. Victory seems so far away. But that is what I pray for, victory over this sin. It cannot happen again like it has in my past. I ask in Jesus Name and for Your sake, Amen.

(24)

I Could Worry Myself Sick

I can worry myself sick about an event coming up or someone that needs help. Worry is the opposite of faith in prayer. When I pray, I do not have to worry, but I tend to worry. In the past I would stay up at night worrying about things or people in my life. Then I learned Psalm chapter one while I was at Jen's house. If I start worrying at night, I meditate on Psalm One or the Twenty-Third Psalm or the LORD's Prayer that Jesus taught His disciples to pray. You cannot worry and think about scripture at the same time.

Be anxious for nothing, but in everything by prayer and supplication, with thanksgiving, let your requests be made known to God; and the peace of God, which surpasses all understanding, will guard your hearts and minds through Christ Jesus. Philippians 4:6-7 (NKJV)

Finally, brethren, whatever things are true, whatever things are noble, whatever things are just, whatever things are pure, whatever things are lovely, whatever things are of good report if there is any virtue and if there is anything praiseworthy—meditate on these things. The things which you learned and received and heard and saw in me, these do, and the God of peace will be with you. Philippians 4:6-9 (NKJV)

Worry and anxiety go hand and hand because I do not put it into the Father's hands. Days when I do not have time to pray and read God's word first thing in the morning cause anxiety in me. I have got to start out my day in God's presence.

"Therefore I say to you, do not worry about your life, what you will eat or what you will drink; nor about your body, what you will put on. Is not life more than food and the body more than clothing? Look at the birds of the air, for they neither sow nor reap nor gather into barns; yet your heavenly Father feeds them. Are you not of more value than they? Which of you by worrying can add one cubit to his stature? "So why do you worry about clothing? Consider the lilies of the field, how they grow: they neither toil nor spin; and yet I say to you that even Solomon in all his glory was not arrayed like one of these. Now if God so clothes the grass of the field, which today is, and tomorrow is thrown into the oven, will He not much more clothe you, O you of little faith? Therefore do not worry, saying, 'What shall we eat?' or 'What shall we drink?' or 'What shall we wear?' For after all these things the Gentiles seek. For your heavenly Father knows that you need all these things. But seek first the kingdom of God and His righteousness, and all these things shall be added to you. Therefore do not worry about tomorrow, for tomorrow will worry about its own things. Sufficient for the day is its own trouble. Matthew 6:25-34 (NKJV)

Worry and anxiety keep me up at night. I take Zeprexa at night to sleep. But I also call Jay, my son, and talk to him in Okinawa where it is day time there when it is night time here. Sometimes I pray. Sometimes I meditate on Psalms 1:1-4, (that is all I have memorized of chapter one of Psalms)

Blessed is the man who walks not in the counsel of the ungodly, Nor stands in the path of sinners, Nor sits in the seat of the scornful; But his delight is in the law of the LORD, And in His law he meditates day and night. He shall be like a tree Planted by the rivers of water, That brings forth its fruit in its season, Whose leaf also shall not wither; and whatever he does shall prosper. The ungodly are not so, But are like the chaff which the wind drives away. Therefore the ungodly shall not stand in the judgment, Nor sinners in the congregation of the righteous. For the LORD knows the way of the righteous, but the way of the ungodly shall perish. Psalm 1:1-6 (NKJV)

Abba, worry and anxiety can make me sick; it is sin sick because worry and anxiety is sin. It is the opposite of peace. God, You are in control. You are not worried about anything. All the people in the world and You are not worried. Do you get rid of worry and anxiety by the fruit of the Spirit called self-control or is it peace? You have concern for us, You did not want us to eat of the tree of life in the Garden of Eden and be able to live forever in our sin. You were concerned enough to put angels at the entrance of the Garden of Eden so no one could ever go back in.

So He drove out the man; and He placed cherubim at the east of the garden of Eden, and a flaming sword which turned every way, to guard the way to the tree of life. Genesis 3:24 (NKJV)

The garden of Eden was a perfect place where Adam and Eve walked with God and talked with God in the cool of the day, until they sinned. We are conceived and born in sin because of Adam. God said Adam would die if he ate of the fruit from the tree of knowledge of good and evil. After Adam ate the forbidden fruit he died spiritually right away. God no longer walked and talked with him. Adam was not allowed to live in the Garden of Eden. He did not die physically at that time. But if you notice in the Bible the words "and he died" you will see it there over and over again all through the Bible. Adam passed his sin nature down to us and we die because of Adam's sin nature. God does not want us to live forever in sin so we die. Jesus is the new Adam and Jesus passes down His Righteousness to the saved. You see, God needed a sacrifice for yours and my sin. In the Old Testament it was bulls, sheep, goats and doves, but it was never enough. It did not solve the sin problem. So in the New Testament of the Bible, Jesus was born to a virgin, God's own Son. He was sinless, not one sin. Jesus was the sacrifice God had been waiting for. Jesus was the perfect Lamb prepared before the foundation of the world. When God made Adam from the dust of the ground, God had already planned and decided Jesus; His only begotten Son would have to be sacrificed on the cross to pay for my sins and your sins. If you will only trust Jesus to save you He will. If you ask God to forgive you in Jesus Name He will. He will let You into Heaven because of the bloodshed by Jesus on the cross. It is enough, Jesus is enough.

Abba, You flooded the earth with water and only saved Noah and his wife and his sons and their wives.

> *Then the LORD saw that the wickedness of man was great in the earth, and that every intent of the thoughts of his heart was only evil continually. And the LORD was sorry that He had made man on the earth, and He was grieved in His heart. So the LORD said, "I will destroy man whom I have created from the face of the earth, both man and beast, creeping thing and birds of the air, for I am sorry that I have made them." But Noah found grace in the eyes of the LORD. This is the genealogy of Noah. Noah was a just man perfect in his generations. Noah walked with God. And Noah begot three sons: Shem, Ham, and Japheth. Genesis 6:5-10 (NKJV)*

And God said to Noah, "The end of all flesh has come before Me, for the earth is filled with violence through them; and behold, I will destroy them with the earth. Make yourself an ark of gopherwood; make rooms in the ark, and cover it inside and outside with pitch. Genesis 6:13-14 (NKJV)

And behold, I Myself am bringing floodwaters on the earth, to destroy from under heaven all flesh in which is the breath of life; everything that is on the earth shall die. Genesis 6:17 (NKJV)

Thus Noah did; according to all that God commanded him, so he did. Then the LORD said to Noah, "Come into the ark, you and all your household, because I have seen that you are righteous before Me in this generation. You shall take with you seven each of every clean animal, a male and his female; two each of animals that are unclean, a male and his female; also seven each of the birds of the air, male and female, to keep the species alive on the face of all the earth. For after seven more days I will cause it to rain on the earth forty days and forty nights, and I will destroy from the face of the earth all living things that I have made." And Noah did according to all that the LORD commanded him. Noah was six hundred years old when the floodwaters were on the earth. So Noah, with his sons, his wife, and his sons' wives, went into the ark because of the waters of the flood. Genesis 6:22and7:1-7 (NKJV)

And God shut the door.

God cared enough for us He sent His own Son—Jesus and He did it right—He never sinned and He died for us so if we believe in Jesus—If we have a relationship with Him and trust Him to save us—we can live forever with God. Eternity starts the moment we are saved.

For God so loved the world that He gave His only begotten Son, that whoever believes in Him should not perish but have everlasting life. For God did not send His Son into the world to condemn the world but that the world through Him might be saved. John 3:16-17 (NKJV)

Now then, we are ambassadors for Christ, as though God were pleading through us: we implore you on Christ's behalf, be reconciled to God. For He made Him who knew no sin to be sin for us, that we might become the righteousness of God in Him. 2 Corinthians 5:20-21 (NKJV)

Abba, forgive me for worrying. It does not do any good to worry and it can do a lot of harm and it keeps me up at night. Thank You for prayer. Thank You that I can talk to You about my concerns and You can do something about my problems. Thank You that when we confess sins to You, You forgive sins. I praise You, You are the best. Your promises are true.

Abba, Father, I pray for a new beginning, like Noah and his sons and their wives. Not a do over—a new life. I want a life without worry and anxiety. I pray for a peace that surpasses all understanding. Help me rely on You, Abba. I love telling You my concerns because You not only are a very good listener— You can do something about my problems when I bring them to You. And even in telling You and asking You for help even when I do not know how to tell You how to help—You help. It helps just to talk to You. It helps just to be in Your presence. Forgive me for worrying and my anxieties. No buts. I send them back up into Your hands, Your capable hands to defuse the problems. I rest in You, obediently. I need Your help to not worry but to pray and meditate on You and on Your Word. I do not have anyone to go watch play sports—I do not watch TV. I have got to talk to You, God. In Jesus Name, Amen.

(25)

Anger Turned Inward Leads to Depression

*A*bba, my first response to any criticism is a response of defensiveness, usually angry defense. Forgive me; help me take constructive criticism and apply it and learn to be better because of it. Help defuse the anger. The kitchen committee is trying to make things easier and better at the same time. Help me grow sensitive to Your leading, Abba. Show me how to change and obey You in the process. Help me smile and laugh at myself. Help me learn by my mistakes or even by others' mistakes so I do not have to go through the same thing they did. I ask in the most Precious Name I know, the Name of Jesus. Amen.

———————————

I get angry with Momma and Daddy when I am told what to do. A lot of the time it is just in my head that I am told what to do. My thoughts of how they have reacted in the past echo in my mind. I have a problem going to them and talking out the problem. I need to talk to them and I do not. Daddy thinks when I talk back to him that I am mad at him. Daddy thinks I am mad at him all the time. I have a very gruff voice and it comes across that way. How I talk and respond makes a difference in how others respond to me. I have learned if I give a smile to someone who does not have one, they usually smile back at me.

When I get mad, I am not nice for a while. I may not cook meals or wash dishes or pick up after myself. I may not talk for a while — a long while. I go to bed angry and with angry conversation going on in my head. By going to bed angry day after day, it leads to depression. I am like a bomb going off that no one can see until it makes me sick. I have learned I can vent that anger to God. God can handle my anger. He even encourages me to vent to Him. Yesterday at the catfish restaurant with Jeff, a week's worth of anger was defused with two sentences. I said, "Spare the rod and spoil the child." Jeff said, "My Dad only knew that one verse of the Bible, and he used it every time he took a buckle to me when I got spanked." I said, "But there is a difference in you and your dad — that is not the only scripture you know, Jeff." He said, "Thank you, Carol." With a few words the point was made and the anger was dissolved.

I know this sin as passive aggression. I am not argumentative. I just plant my feet firmly and I just do not do it. Forgive me; I do it to You too, God. This has been my homework assignment since 7-18-08: to write down my sins You showed me and their consequences. I have read what I am supposed to do in *Downpour* by James MacDonald. I have wanted to go on to the next chapter that teaches repentance, but I did not want to deal with the sin in my life, especially this much of it. It seemed overwhelming to me. If I am lukewarm, God will spit me out of His mouth. I do not want to be spit out. I do not want to be lukewarm. That is why I read the *Downpour* book. I wanted revival, but there was so much sin in me. I would not finish reading it until I dealt with my sins. Repentance! That is what has to happen before there can be a downpour in my life.

But nothing has overwhelmed me more than the feeling of heaviness over my life. It was not until You spoke to me and told me I am already forgiven of those sins that I have agreed to go on and do this homework assignment. Not guilty is written all over my sins. I tore some of the pages out and shredded them. I had used a black Sharpie to mark out some of the things written. As I shredded them You whispered over me, **"It is under the blood, under the blood, under the blood of Jesus."** Abba, I want everything else under the blood of Jesus too, all my sins. I agree with You to do what You ask me.

Anger turned inward leads to depression and makes me sick emotionally. And it does not do good things for my relationship with Momma and Daddy. I was quick to bring up past sins and how people had hurt me in the past. My response was you never do this or you always do that. It would not just be the thing going on right at the moment. I would dredge up all the old times someone disappointed me or that person hurt me in some way. I would get angry inside and pent up anger leads to depression. It is like a time bomb waiting to go off, either attacking me on the inside or me blowing up at someone else.

If I do not forgive others, God does not forgive me. Hate is a strong word, but unforgiveness can build to hate.

God showed me what sin looks like. There was a smell on our back porch two different times this summer of 2008. The smell got so bad; we started looking to see what the cause was. Two different times we found that a cat had died, and they were unrecognizable. Maggots had completely eaten away at the body until it did not even look like a cat anymore. Maggots were everywhere in the body cavity. Teeming and moving and eating away. We had to clean up that mess. We had to get close to do it. The smell was death. Once you've smelled death, you do not forget. Sin is like carrying around a dead body on your back. I am not talking about a recently dead body like the movie, Weekend at Bernie's. I am talking about the dead body full of the maggots and the stench and the smell of death. Sin will eventually kill you, and without Jesus in your life God has no alternative but for you to go to

Hell. Not asking God to forgive you is a sin. Unbelief is a sin. It only takes this one sin for you not to be saved. Every word of the Bible is true. I did not believe that for a long time but I now know the Bible is all true.

(26)

Healthy Ways to Vent

*T*alk it over with God on a long walk and use up all the emotion.

Talk to the person you are angry with and tell them why you are angry. Acknowledge their feelings too. I cannot do anything about their anger but I can do something about my anger.

Do not go to bed angry. Do not let the sun go down on your wrath. Deal with anger daily. Do not let it build from day to day—week to week–month to month or even year to year. Today is the day to do something about the anger before it smolders and starts a chemical reaction in my brain or a heart problem of unforgiveness or an angry reaction I will regret later.

I need to forgive because I have been forgiven a lot.

Do not drag up the past. Deal with the present. You cannot say "You always do this" or "You never do that." Just deal with the issue at hand today. Do not curse God and die. That is what Job's wife told him to do; that is what Satan wants you to do.

God, You say in the Bible,

> *"Be angry, and do not sin": do not let the sun go down on your wrath nor give place to the devil.* Ephesians 4:26 (NKJV)

Jesus, You did not get angry when we crucified You. You forgave. You got angry in the temple. Why? What is the difference? One, the temple where God abode on earth, the other, the Temple of the Holy Spirit—God in the flesh. I know it is okay to be angry with You, You not only allow it, You encourage it. You want us to voice our anger and put it into words to You. You can handle our anger. Abba, most people do not know I get angry, but You know—I can hide nothing from You. Thank You that it is that way. In Jesus Name, Amen.

Search me, O God, and know my heart; Try me, and know my anxieties; And see if there is any wicked way in me, And lead me in the way everlasting. Psalm 139:23-24 (NKJV)

Abba, I do not curse any more out loud. Thank You and I praise You. But when I get angry, and I let it smolder and when I do not deal with it, I still think curse words. Forgive me, Jesus. I do not want to curse even in my thoughts. Help me deal with anger and passive aggression in a healthy way, in a godly way and in a way that glorifies You, Jesus. Help me with the daily-ness of sin, so I can confess it to You and accept Your forgiveness. Forgive me, cleanse me, heal me, revive me and restore unto me the fellowship of Thy Holy Spirit. Restore unto me the joy of Thy salvation.

Father, please forgive me for unforgiveness. It does not matter to Carolyn if someone does not like her. She just tries to love them into loving her. Help me forgive them. Help me love them until they love me too. Forgive me and help me forgive quickly and completely. It does not matter what they did; help my response be to forgive them, and love them. You forgive me, and because of that, my response should be forgiveness. Forgive me my trespasses as I forgive those who trespass against me. Forgive me for both pride and pretentiousness. I want to be like You, Father. I want to be the very image of Christ. I need Your help. Pride puffs me up, and makes me feel more important than I am. I like it when people say good things about me.

Abba, I need Your help, I need Your forgiveness. I need to see Your way is better. Help me talk out my frustrations and anger instead of it being a smoldering bomb waiting to detonate into either an explosion onto other people or a chemical warfare in my brain, leading to depression or passive aggression aimed at someone else. I turn away from this sin of anger and of my way of showing it to Your way. You got angry, but you did not sin when You got angry. Teach me Your way of anger management—a holy and righteous anger that can be expressed and dealt with. Help me bring my anger to You first and sift it through Your love and counsel before I blow up at someone and lash out at them. Help me talk to them and not someone else—not gossip—but take it to the person I am having the problem with. Teach me, forgive me, cleanse me, heal me, and restore unto me the joy of Thy salvation. This is a life of habit—this is how I have always handled it. I would get angry until it made me physically or emotionally sick. It is not an option now—You have shown me a better way. There is no way out of this except through the cross.

(27)

Adopted by God

April Thursday 4-3-08

*A*bba, Father, I want a holy fear of You, God, I run to You. You adopted me into Your family. Now I have the best of both. I still belong to my family here on earth, and I have been adopted into God's family in heaven. Thank you for listening. You can do something about my problems.

I have always bailed out of my jobs and quit because I did not like being told what to do. I did not like that authority over me. I would last about three years at a job before I could not handle it anymore, and I would quit. It has happened over and over again and then I would change jobs and go to a new boss. I do not like being told what to do. But what about You, God, You are the authority over me, You tell me what to do. Do I do it to you, too?

Abba, Forgive me over and over again. I resent people who are in authority over me. Help me with other people, but I am also concerned about my relationship with You. I do not want to resent Your authority over me. I want to obey You because You deserve obedience. I want You to tell me what to do. Help me never resent You or my boss ever again. I pray to love and meet needs just like You love and meet my needs. Forgive me.

Is that why I left the missions organization where I was volunteering? I was to the point I did not like being told what to do, but Bro. Bill was right. If he asked me to do something a certain way, he had a good reason for doing it that way. I did not always argue with him, but my passive aggression would kick in, and I was not doing my best work. If I was angry, I did not want to talk to him about what was the problem. Was I just in rebellion to his authority over me? I wanted to be able to do the job my way.

Abba, forgive me for my rebellion to the authority You have placed over me. Forgive me ultimately for my rebellion to Your authority over me. Bro. Randy is my authority over me. When I am at the mission organization, Bro. Bill is the authority over me. Daddy and Momma are the authority over me at home.

Help me! Help me! Help me! I pray to grow spiritually through this. Help me conform to Your Word. I pray for godly wisdom, godly understanding, godly knowledge, godly revelation, godly discernment and sound judgment to grace my neck. I pray to see it from Your point of view, to see Your role, Your rule and Your reign. I pray to see where I am in this picture. I pray to see man's role. I pray to see God's role. I pray for Your help, and I pray for Your grace, tender mercies and loving kindnesses. I do not want to quit this time. I pray for victory in Christ over this sin in my life. I surrender to Your will, I submit to Your authority over me, and I pray You will sanctify me. I pray for self control by Your Holy Spirit's power to Your honor, glory and praise. Thank You and I praise You. I love You, and I want the whole world to know that I love You by the way I love them.

Abba, I worked some Wednesday for the fellowship supper, but Tracy and Al did the work. I need Your help. I do not know where my pay check is and I need to deposit it so I can pay Tracie for all her help for the time she worked while I was resting. Father God, please let the scales fall from my eyes that I may see, even as You see, where it is. You know where it is. God, would You please show me where I put the paycheck. In the Holy Name of my Jesus, Amen. I found the check, but when I told Tracie what I was going to pay her, she said I did not have to do that. I praise God for showing me where my paycheck was.

Bro. Bill let me drive Mary's van. I took it back to him when I got bad around spring break. Bro. Randy let me drive his car. I cannot really remember how long I drove the little white car, but when Bro. Randy needed it back, Bro. Bill again let me drive Mary's van. Bro. Bill gave the keys to the office back to me as well as the cell phone even though I did not go back to work for him. The LORD gives and the LORD takes away. Blessed be the Name of the LORD and then the LORD gave again. I praise God because Bro. Bill let me drive the van again.

(28)

Pride and Gossip

*A*bba, forgive me for my foolish pride. I pray for a spirit of humility. Keep me humble. Forgive me, cleanse me, heal me, restore me to a right spirit with You and restore unto me Your full measure of joy. I may not brag to other people, but I think more highly of myself than I ought. What You do through me should be to Your glory not mine. I miss out on giving God the glory if I take it for myself. Pride goes before a fall. Forgive me for my pride that puffs me up and gives me an important spirit. It is just a smoke screen because when it is blown away I am not much. Holy Spirit fill all the holes, where my pride was, with Your Spirit. I need You. I cannot do this on my own. I know what I am like, and it is not pretty. Forgive me and thank You I do not have to have a dominating spirit. Fill all the hollow places; this forgiven sin leaves, with Your Holy Spirit. Fill me completely and to overflowing with Your Holly Spirit. I need Your forgiveness and Your relationship. I love You, I glorify You, I honor You, and I hold You high and lifted up. I praise You, Halleluiah! I am so in awe of You—I adore You. Knowing You is the best thing that has ever happened to me. You help me so much on Wednesdays when I cook—help me give You the credit. I could not do it without You. I pray to lift You up instead of myself. The only way I am important is

Christ's importance in me. Let me point people to You, LORD. I pray to be humble, meek and gentle just like You, Jesus.

Abba, if I gossip with one person she will think I will gossip about her. Most stories are best left unsaid and just prayed about. Sometimes I would tell something on the pretense that it was a prayer request, but I should have just prayed about it and not told anyone else. I got in so much trouble with this one, LORD that Momma and Daddy will not even talk in front of me anymore. I am sorry. Please put a watch guard on my mouth. Please forgive me; gossip serves no purpose in and of itself. It only cuts down other people. Help me not to gossip and help me not to listen to gossip. Help me pray about problems instead of talking about people and events. People tell me things in strictest confidence. I have to keep it that way. If I do not, they are not going to trust me. Help me, Abba to remember what things are just between You and me. Let it not go any further than that. You, God, listen to every word spoken and unspoken. LORD, teach us to pray about and for other people. If we just talk about someone or something, it serves no purpose. But teach us to stop right then and pray about the situation before it turns into gossip. Gossip tears down people, and I want to build them up and encourage them in You, LORD. Thank You for forgiving me. Please put a watch guard on me, my mind and my tongue that I will not gossip any more.

Abba, years ago You showed me that it is almost impossible to stop gossip once it gets started. You showed me that with some styrofoam packing peanuts that blew outside and scattered over the yard. I knew it was my responsibility to pick them all up. Thank You that the wind was not blowing or it would have been impossible to do. But it was hard and it took a lot of time. Help me not to spread rumors to the four winds. Help me speak the truth in love. Help me stop the wildfire of gossip by simply letting it die with me and never repeating it to anyone else. Help me not to listen to gossip, but God, help me to pray and bring the problem to You right then. You hear us, help us voice our concerns by talking and listening to You, because You not only listen to our prayers, You do something about them. Help us see Your answer as the answer to our prayers. I am bossy in the kitchen at church. I want it done my way, but my way is too hard even for a team of cooks. I could lose my help. I could lose my friends. I could lose my job. I make cooking in the kitchen at church much harder than it should be. Abba, maybe there is pride attached to this sin, too. I do things by the recipe. I do things the way I have always done it. I do not listen to others' advice. Forgive me and help them forgive me for how I have acted in the past. Help me listen to wise counsel from Al, Tracie, and the Kitchen Committee. They are trying to make things easier and better at the same time. Help me grow sensitive to Your leading, Abba. Show me how to change and obey You in the process. Help me smile and laugh at myself. Help me learn by my mistakes or even by other's mistakes so I do not have to go through the same thing they did.

I have learned I do not like being told what to do. It goes against every fiber of my being. I want to do what I want to do. And, therefore, that is SIN. Notice the I in the middle of the word SIN. SIN is doing whatever I want to do instead of what God wants me to do. I cannot think, say, or do what I want to do just because I always did it that way. I have to change. I have to stay on the budget and change the way I cook. Now I am told what I can and cannot do. But it has been good. It is not so bad being on a budget and it is easier to fix meals now.

"Simplify recipes
    Simplify meals
        Simplify ingredients
            Wing it sometimes
                Healthy meals
                    Colorful meals
                        Variety
                            Get out of the rut
                                Do not make it so hard."
In Jesus Name, Amen

God spoke,
"Smile and have a good time".

111

(29)

Dancing With the Angels

September Saturday 9-13-08

*A*bba, I talked with Robyn about being an understudy to the angels who dance and do motions during the Christmas program this year at church. She said I could. Help me. LORD continue to teach me to dance. Help me dance even if it is for You alone I dance. I pray You will continue to refine the motions of the angels. I pray we will have balance as we learn and at each night of the presentation, working, playing, loving, and resting as needed. I pray for the angels that they will be healthy and well, so I do not have to take their place. Thank You, I get to dance for You. I am also in charge of props so help me be ready with whatever is needed this year. Help us with the crowns — not only the halos the angels wear, but also the crowns the kings wear and Jesus' crown. I pray for the choir as the participating churches come together. Help us with the music. This year we are doing the best of the best of all twelve years we have been doing the living singing Christmas tree. Thank You, we are not doing the Christmas tree this year. We are doing something better, "A Street in Bethlehem. I praise You and thank You in advance for all the lives You will touch through the program. Please save people who come. Help us introduce lost people to Jesus, I ask it according to Your will.

Abba, I am learning to dance with the angels, who will be participating in the Christmas program at church, during practice on Sunday afternoons. I did not want to get up in front of the choir Wednesday night to practice. I was so unsure of myself. I do not even know if it was my idea or Yours? Do I continue? I am just an understudy just in case something happens to another angel and I have to do it. I have about two months to learn it. Help me. LORD, dance and sing and smile through me — I cannot remember the songs, words and moves. Can You do that through me? Diane stayed late after choir practice and helped me learn some more, but the remedial angel practice is on Wednesday nights after Fellowship supper, while I am still cleaning up the kitchen. When am I supposed to practice with them? I pray for freedom. I pray for peace that passes all understanding. I pray for Your Holy Presence in me. I pray to be secure in You. I pray to trust You, Abba. Act and react through me. Do You want me to be an angel this year? Teach me to dance. I pray for more angels. I pray for the choir. I cannot afford one hundred dollars for a costume; others may have this problem, too. Please meet this need. I pray for security in Jesus. I pray to dance for You—to Your glory and honor and praise. I confess my inhibition and insecurity to You.

Thank You, Abba, I did not dance at the Christmas program, but I thank You for the opportunity to try. Thank You for Cindy and how she stepped in and took Penny's place.Thank You for Robyn's and the other angel's patience with me.

Abba. Please forgive me, I need You to show up and be big in me. Less of me and a whole lot more of You, Jesus. I need You to go with me to new places and to meet new people. Bro. Randy talked about a tapestry this past Sunday in the sermon. He said we see our life as all the loose pieces of string on the wrong side of a tapestry. It is dark, dull, and ugly until You weave Yourselves, Abba, Jesus and Holy Spirit into our lives and into our tapestries. Help me see it from Your perspective. Help me see the front side of the tapestry, the finished side. I give You my permission to do whatever You want to finish me and complete me. I want to see my life from the right side and not the wrong side.

Jesus, I do not try things that are new. I do not try what I know I cannot do. Therefore, I am unable to do a lot of new things. I do not go to places I have never been before unless I am with someone else. Insecurity disables me in trying a lot of different things and going to a lot of different places. I did not like being alone, and sometimes I felt the loneliest when I was in a crowd. If I do not reach out to others, they will not reach in to me. If I do not reach out to others, I am alone in this world.

Abba, I could stay alone with You in my room all day and all night and be happy. I resent people intruding on my time with God. But I could spend all day with You and it still would not be enough. I miss out on other people if I resent their intrusions of my time with God. Forgive me.

You have a world of people out there for me to meet. Help me touch lives and be touched by others. Help me see the need of having other people in my life. People are important to You; make them as important to me as they are to You. Help me be a friend to someone who needs a friend today. Help me talk with others and see their problems and concerns as important. Help me care for others. Help me want to love and meet their needs. Help me do better than I have done in the past. I pray others will know how much I love You by how much I love them. I need Your help and I need a downpour of Your Holy Spirit. Forgive me for being such a loner. Thank You and I praise You. I ask in my precious Jesus' Name, Amen.

(30)

Bitter or Better?

$\mathcal{M}$y consequences were that I hurt myself, and I overflow bitterness onto other people around me. It is my
choice. I choose better!

Abba, forgive me for all the times before when I did not
choose better, and I chose to be very bitter. I do not want to
be hard and bitter about my life. It is a gift from You. Help me
unwrap it day by day. You promise nothing more than what
I can handle as long as I allow You to handle it, handle it,
handle it. I try to not pick it back up and carry the load that
has always been reserved for You. I choose to get better, by
depending on You. In Jesus Name, Amen.

But even with the reduced work load, I did not get better.
The people at church continued to pray for me. I met with Bro.
Randy and told him I was having problems. He got me in touch
with a Christian counseling center in north central Texas. I
learned from them I did not have the right Medicare-Medicaid
to be able to pay to see a doctor. Several weeks went by. I
had a procedure done at the hospital and told Sherry, who
works there, of my predicament. She looked up my Medicare
and Medicaid information. I had everything I needed including
Part A and Part B. So next time I was in town I had Momma
take me by the Christian counseling office. The receptionist

there still told me I did not have the right stuff to see the doctors there.

BUT God!

Then the receptionist said a new psychologist had just started working there who accepted patients who only had Medicare or Medicaid or whatever they thought I had to pay for it. So an appointment was made for me to see Dr. Snowden on July 1, 2008.

(31)

A Cracked Vessel

*I*n the meantime I started meeting with Bro. Randy, my Pastor and his wife, Pam for counseling. Pam taught me something she learned from Ruth Fellowship Ministries that sometimes God takes our broken vessels and picks up all the broken pieces and starts putting us back together. But since He is the Master Potter and we are just clay in His hands, He has the prerogative to put our broken pieces of clay (our lives) and put them back together with cracks still in places. I had always thought when God molded us he was working with soft clay. But with me he had hard clay, and the pieces did not quite fit back together again even looking like a pot, but God does not make junk.

God started asking me to walk with Him in the cool of the day; summers can be very hot in my hometown. So to avoid the sun I walked at sunrise and sunset. God started showing me how beautiful it was when Jesus could shine through the cracks of my life. He started by showing me sunrises and sunsets where there were trees in the way of actually seeing the sun. I only got glimpses of the sun through the open places between the leaves. Then God showed me sunrises where there were clouds and I only got to see the sun for only a few seconds or minutes depending on the cloud formations. Then God showed me how beautiful a sunrise is when it is all clouds below but we can still see the glow of the sun, like a silver lining. God showed me a sunrise where the sun came up from behind the clouds and all around me on all sides the sun shone and reflected on all the other clouds. My favorite way of seeing the sun is when the clouds are scattered and the sun beams shine all the way to the ground. So I started asking God to shine through my cracks. It has been raining. The Son is still shining. We have been praying for rain here where I live. God sends the rain. I praise Him for every drop. One day the clouds were overcast, so I got to walk longer than usual. You see my medication made me allergic to the sun. So that is why I started walking at sunrise and sunset. But this day it was completely cloudy. So I kept on walking. The sun burned off all the clouds that day. Jesus can do that in our lives too, if we will let Him.

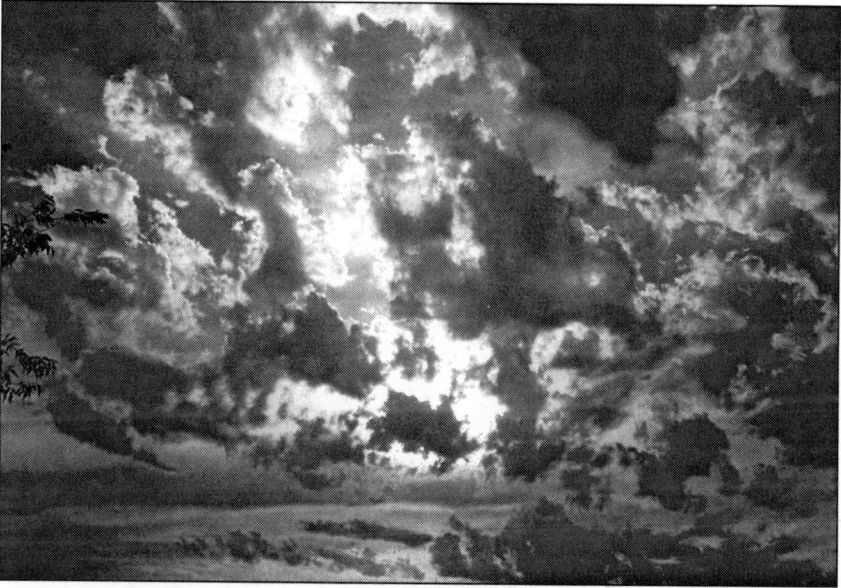

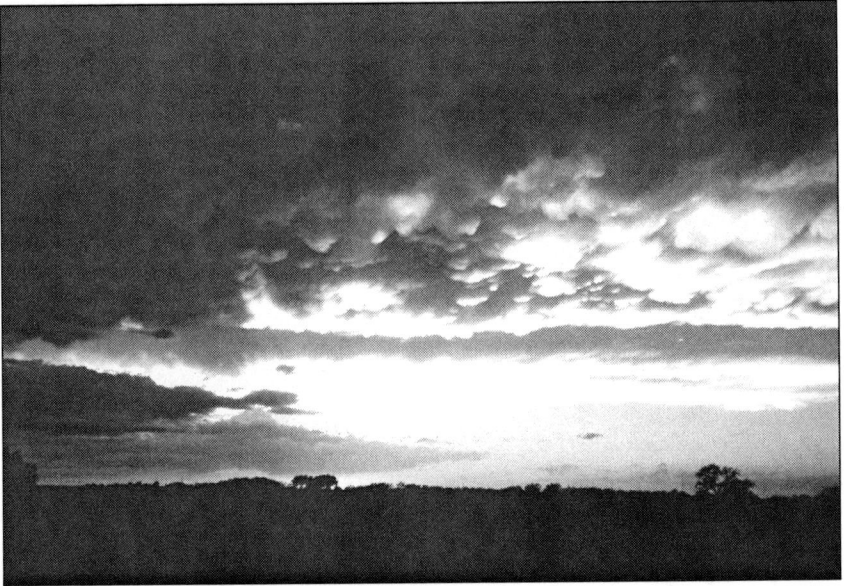

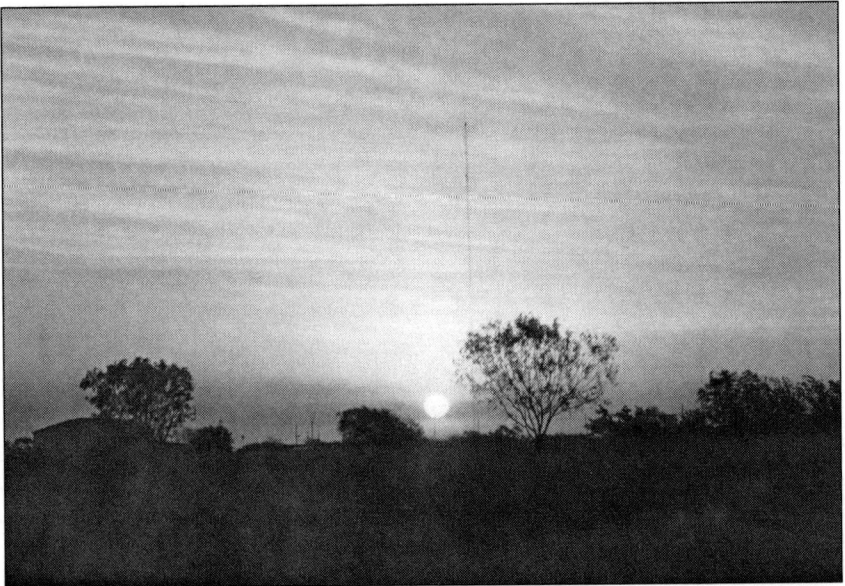

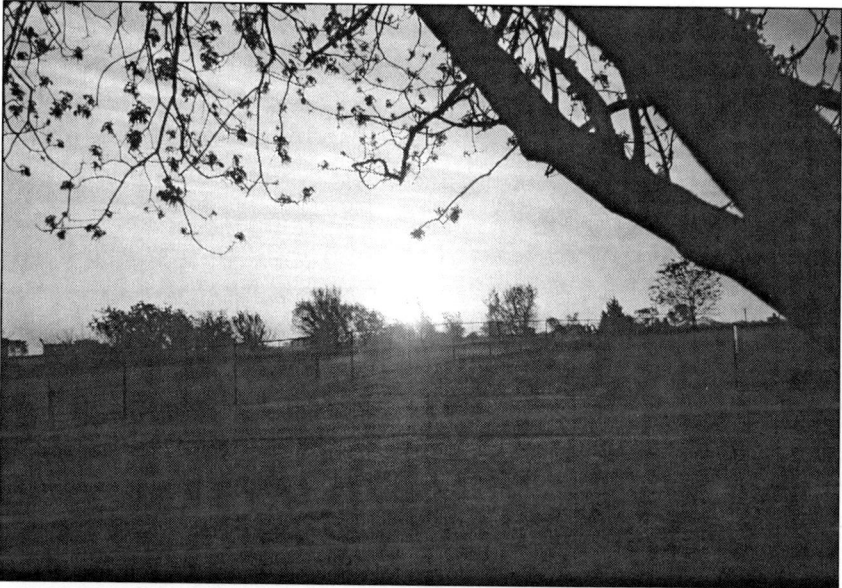

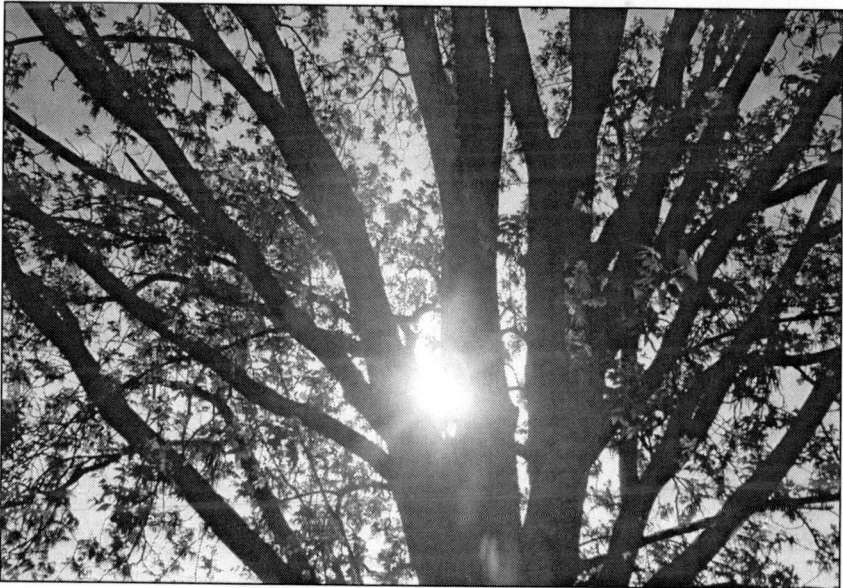

Monday, August 18, 2008

I was having my quiet time with God, and I heard the rain. As I went to the door, I was disappointed that I would not get to walk that day. But God! God asked me to step out in the rain. I felt the rain on me. God touched me with the rain. I lifted my head and hands and praised Him. My eyes were closed. Then I opened my eyes, and God showed me the light still there even on a very cloudy day shining ever so gently through the leaves of the pecan trees at my front door. Clouds may come, but they do not have to get us down. God is Faithful. God is good all the time through good days and even and especially in dark days when He is closer than we can even understand and very active in our lives behind the scenes of what we can see with our eyes. Would you ask God to shine through you?

When Jen got married, I was sitting on the second row in the church. The flower girl took her basket of petals and poured all of the flower petals at the bottom of the steps up to the stage. When Jen walked up the steps, the flower petals bubbled up through the cut work of the train of her dress. It was so beautiful and I do not think anyone else saw it. I want God's Holy Spirit to bubble out of me through all those cracks God has left in me on purpose.

May Saturday 5-31-08

God, three in one, the Holy Trinity, I walked with You this morning. You were so quiet. You listened to my heart and to my words. You provided a horse for me to pet and a black and white dog to protect me from the other two dogs. Thank You. You provided a sunrise to see through the leaves so I could see how You God can shine through the cracks. I am broken before You God, imperfect in all my ways compared to You God. But God You are putting me back together. Shine through the cracks in me, Your broken vessel. Fill me full and overflowing with Your Holy Spirit. Forgive me for loving another. And tune my heart once again to respond to Your love, to You alone my love, my Jesus.

God spoke, "**God may be invisible to you right now but I am not absent.**"

> *Love suffers long and is kind; love does not envy; love does not parade itself, is not puffed up; does not behave rudely, does not seek its own, is not provoked, thinks no evil; does not rejoice in iniquity, but rejoices in the truth; bears all things, believes all things, hopes all things, endures all things. Love never fails.* 1 Corinthians 13:4-8A (NKJV)

God, You are not distant; You are able to touch, You are very present, You are powerful in our lives. You are vocal, You are listening, You are active in our lives, and You are working and praying and answering behind the scenes. Even when we cannot see You, You are seeing us. You are there in Heaven and here with me at the same time. You are patient, You are kind, You are long suffering, You are selfless, You are self sacrificing, Your love is not dormant, You are agape love, and I need Your agape love, God, in me. Fill me with the Holy Spirit's agape love for all others but especially for Jesus and You, Heavenly Father. Jesus suffers long, so empower me to suffer long. He is kind, so let me be kind. You do not parade Yourself, so I pray I will not either, Your love is not puffed up, please do not let mine be puffed up either. Your love does not behave rudely; therefore, please do not let Your love in me behave rudely either. Help me not to seek my own way, help me not to provoke. I pray I will not think evil thoughts. I pray I will not rejoice in iniquity, but that I will rejoice in Your truth. I pray to bear all things, believe all things, hope all things, and endure all things. Love never fails. May the love You fill me with never fail to love others as You have loved me and to love Jesus, my Husband to be. Forgive me for getting my eyes on another. Jesus, my big Brother, You never fail. I ask for Jesus sake and for His glory and in His Name, Amen.

June Wednesday 6-11-08

Abba Father, Jesus, Holy Spirit, thank You for time off. Thank You for all the pain. It brought me to the Holy Trinity of You, God. Thank You for all the confusion. It makes me seek Your face and Your will for my life. Thank You for the clouds of depression; it will not be like this forever — one day — one day heaven will be reality and I will never feel like this again. Thank You for today, a day of promise and new starts. Thank You that You walk with me in the valley of the shadow of death. Thank You for Momma, Daddy, Nanny, Jen, Jeff, Mackenzie, Lena, Jay, Melissa, Garrett and Colby. Even if I cannot see my children and grandchildren all the time, they are still there. Immanuel means God with us. Thank You; You are still very much God with us even, and especially when we cannot see You. Thank You for food in the ice box and freezer, and cooking and cleaning and the dishwasher, washer, dryer, oven, stove and microwave oven. Thank You that we are alive, alive more than ever before because Christ lives in us. Thank You for Buh, Jan, Debbie, Paula, Trudy, Jason and Shawn. Please save them and please save Lena and Garrett and Colby, too. Thank You for saving Mackenzie. Thank You for Bryan, Dewayne, Cindy, Lisa, Carol, and all my family.

Thank You for dark days. Thank You that You can shine brighter in dark days. Please, shine through me. Jesus shine through the cracks just like Pam, taught me, Jesus shine through the cracks You left in me on purpose. God truly is the potter and we are just the clay. I am hard, and twisted and broken as the song says. Break me more, if needed, God as long as I can be Your mosaic piece of art in Your hands, fashioned by the Master potter's hands. Thank You that You break me. Thank You that You can put me back together better than before; better than I could have ever imagined or dreamed. Thank You for Pam, Bro. Randy, Bro. Jim, Sandra, Bro. Jimmy and Cindy. Thank You, for all of the people at First Baptist Church. Thank You for the lost waiting to hear of Jesus. Let us not disappoint them. Fill me with Your Holy Spirit until Your Spirit overflows through the cracks You left in me on purpose. Thank You and I praise You. I ask in Jesus Christ's Name, Amen.

Vacation Bible School

God called me to teach missions for Vacation Bible School (VBS) this year at First Baptist Church in the same church in which I grew up. And God shone. Tracie and Nancy and I decorated three rooms sometimes staying up very late into the night, I did not stay up as long as they did. We enjoy each other's company, and it was great getting to be together so much. Shelby and Sydney, Tracie's girls, were there sometimes too, and it was great fun. I had always worked with crafts before in VBS, so it was new ground for me to teach missions. I loved teaching missions. We had a mission's outreach project called a party-in-a-box. The kids in VBS collected birthday party supplies to give a birthday party for the kids who might not get to have a birthday otherwise, and we gave the boxes of birthday supplies to the Outreach Mission here in the town I grew up in. The kids made different messages to put in the boxes to tell about Jesus and their testimonies and what they had learned in VBS. I got to read all their messages, and they were great. We learned that missionaries sometimes use storying cloths which have pictures that remind us of Bible stories. Since we cannot talk to the kids in person who will get the party-in-a-box, we included the story of Jesus in written form as well as the storying cloths they had made in class that had pictures to represent the story of Jesus' life.

The Story of Jesus. You too can tell the story of Jesus.

About 2,000 years ago a star in the east led the wise men and shepherds to a stable where they found a baby wrapped in swaddling clothes lying in a manger. His name is Jesus, our Immanuel, which means, God with us.

He is God's own Son. Jesus led a perfect life. He never sinned—not one time. Jesus died on the cross for your sins and mine. So if we trust in Jesus, He can forgive us of our sins if we ask.

Three days after Jesus died on the cross, He came back to life. For forty days He stayed with the people eating with them, teaching them, and helping them to better understand who He was and why He had come. Then in a cloud He went back to Heaven.

Someday in a cloud, He is coming back to take Christians, His church, His bride, back to Heaven with Him.

That is what we sent, just a simple story of Jesus' life.

(33)

Our Vacation

I had to leave Friday morning early, so I could not be at VBS that morning. My daughter and her family were going to go to our family reunion this year in Branson, Missouri. Daddy, Momma and I left Friday morning from Texas and headed that way. Jen, Jeff, Mackenzie and Lena did not leave till Saturday morning to go to Branson. The girls had been in the car all day, and then we immediately went to see *Noah's Ark* at Sights and Sounds Theater. It was so good the kids sat mesmerized, glued to their seats.

I got to go back to Jen and Jeff's house with them on Sunday morning going back to the Illinois side of Saint Louis, Missouri. Because I got to go back home with Jen and her family and stayed for two and a half weeks, I had to reschedule my appointment with Dr. Snowden till July 25th. Before I left to go to Branson and Jen's house, Dr. Wieck, my psychiatrist increased my medicine, but it made me feel like the world was happening around me, but I was not a part of it. It also made me allergic to the sun. So the dosage was decreased as soon as I returned to Texas. I still had a wonderful time with Jen and her family. Mackenzie (Jen's oldest daughter) had been to the same VBS as we had at our church, and so we practiced together the sign language and songs from Outrigger Island that was our VBS theme in 2008. My daughter, Jen, works from home. I kept the dishes loaded in the dishwasher and made sure Jen had sweet iced tea or coffee to drink each day. Lena (Jen's youngest daughter) stayed at day care, but we had time together in the afternoons and evenings and all day long on the weekends. Jeff, Jen's husband, just retired from 20 years in the Air Force. He now works for a bread company in Saint Louis. He kept us stocked with all kinds of different breads and bagels to try. I am so glad I got to stay with them, but I was so confused while I was there. I learned that was a side effect of the medicine. As soon as they brought me back home to Texas, I reduced the medicine I was taking for bipolar back down, with Dr. Wieck's advice, to what I had been taking for the last five years. For five years it had been keeping me fairly level. My highs weren't too high and my lows weren't too low.

July Friday PM 7-25-08

Abba, thank You and I praise You—I have been with Jen, Jeff, Mackenzie and Lena at their house. We met up with them at the family reunion in Branson that weekend before I went to stay with them. The week before I left, Momma taught the smaller kids crafts and I taught missions during Vacation Bible School. Thank You it was a wonderful week with the kids, but because we had to leave early Friday morning to go to Branson, someone else had to take our places for VBS that day. Thank You for the family of God. Please help Kristi get the 6th grade class to teach during the new school year. Please help the Lavys get jobs when they get laid off at work. I pray a special prayer for Crystal—You know what it is about. Draw her close to You. Help her through this time. I pray for Amy, be with her. Help us all get to church on Sundays and Wednesdays. In Jesus Name, Amen.

(34)

Encouraged to Talk

I think Al, Nancy's husband, was the first one to try to convince me to talk about my problems. He has helped me on Wednesday afternoons and evenings to cook for the Fellowship Suppers at the church. Talking comes hard for me. Most every time I cycled to depression I would be silent, sometimes for months. I would not talk to my first psychiatric doctor for years. I would go to see him for visits and we would just sit in silence. I was very sad after the divorce. I just could not get over it. I could not get past it for years and years on end. Even Buh said I just needed to go on with my life. But I did not feel I was living. I felt as if something had died inside of me, and I just could not make it come back to life. I learned that when you go through a divorce, it is like a death—the death of a marriage. It is okay to mourn that death. But my sadness lasted for years. I would not accept that it was God's will for me to be divorced and live just with my children. I held on to God healing my marriage long after the divorce papers were signed, and Buh was remarried. Aunt Sallie showed me a verse in the Bible that spoke to my situation.

> *...then her former husband who divorced her must not take her back to be his wife after she has been defiled; for that is an abomination before the LORD, and you*

shall not bring sin on the land which the LORD your God is giving you as an inheritance. Deuteronomy 24:4 (NKJV)

That settled it in my heart that I was not supposed to be married to Buh even if he got divorced. It was a sin against God to go back to my former husband to marry him again.

I could not let go of the sadness. It had a grip on me. Each time one of my children left home, it became worse. I did not know what to do with myself when they left home, and I finally was all alone.

I fear being alone. Yet for most of my life I was loneliest in a crowd. God had to work on this in me. He has taught me to not look at the crowd as a whole, but to find one person to talk to even if I do not know them. Find out her name because her name is so important to her and try to use her name in the conversation. I have to work at this because my memory is so bad. If you are really interested in her and ask a few questions she will talk to you and with you and the crowd fades into the background.

I do not remember exactly when I came to understand that Jesus, by His Holy Spirit, is with me always. I do not know if I know it enough now to live by myself, even now I live with my parents. I do not have to be by myself very often. I do not know what it will be like when I have to be on my own without them. I have put my name on a list to move into a government apartment by myself. When they call, I will make a decision with God's help to know if I can live alone or not.

Sadness overwhelmed me. It took control of my emotions. Happiness was fleeting or non-existent. It robbed me of the joy of the LORD. I did not get joy until I learned from Beth Moore that joy had been appropriated to me already. That means it has been given to me, but I have to choose joy. It is a gift from God, so now I choose joy over sadness. I choose God's way—joy over sadness and the depression.

Abba, I need fear no one except You. I pray for a holy fear toward You. Not afraid of You but a reverence and awe of who

You really are. Help me with my fear of being alone. Help me with my fear of being left behind when the rapture happens and You come back for Your Bride the church. Forgive me for being afraid. What have I to fear as long as I have You in my life? I was not left behind, the rapture has not really happened, yet. Abba, You speak to me at times when I am alone telling me that You will never leave me nor forsake me. Why is it still fresh? Why does it still hurt? Will You heal me? Will You make it better? LORD, increase my faith in You. Thank You and I praise You for Your presence.

Abba, forgive me for my sadness. Thank You that You make me alive again. You make me want to go on another day. Jesus, You make life worth living again. Thank You for my new life in Christ. But I was in Christ when I was so sad. I am sorry it lasted so long. I am sorry I would not let go of the sadness. Thank You it is gone now. I do not even cry about my divorce anymore. I am not even sure when or why it went away. I just know it is not a sin anymore. Thank You for healing me, Abba, my DADDY. Thank You for Your joy, comfort and peace. Thank You for Your love and support. Thank You Jesus for interceding for me and for all the people who have prayed for me to get well. I praise You I am well. Thank You for healing me. It does not hurt anymore, not at all. I praise You, God. Thank You. In Jesus Blessed Name, Amen.

July Friday PM 7-25-08

I have withdrawn all my life. When I am hurt, I move closer and closer into myself and withdraw inside myself. I will stay inside my room in my house and only go out if I absolutely have to. I withdraw from family and friends and I did not even know or realize that I had withdrawn from God. When I give up on God, I tie His hands in answering my prayers. God is big, and I do not always think of how He is going to answer prayer. I do not think the way God does. He has a perfect plan, and I need to keep in step with Him and do it His way.

Jennifer, from church, is expecting a baby right now. We had her baby shower last Sunday afternoon. She just bubbled. She talked as she opened all the gifts. We had the best time. She is expecting a baby and it brings joy to her heart.

I am expecting good things to come from Your hand to me, Father.

For I know the plans I have for you, says the LORD. They are plans for good and not for evil, to give you a future and a hope. Jeremiah 29:11 (TLB)

And the LORD God said, "It is not good that man should be alone; I will make him a helper comparable to him." Out of the ground the LORD God formed every beast of the field and every bird of the air, and brought them to Adam to see what he would call them. And whatever Adam called each living creature, that was its name. So Adam gave names to all the cattle, to the birds of the air, and to every beast of the field. But for Adam there was not found a helper comparable to him.

And the LORD God caused a deep sleep to fall on Adam, and he slept; and He took one of his ribs, and closed up the flesh in its place. Then the rib which the LORD God had taken from man He made into a woman, and He brought her to the man. And Adam said: "This is now bone of my bones And flesh of my flesh; She shall be called Woman, Because she was taken out of Man." Therefore a man shall leave his father and mother and be joined to his wife, and they shall become one flesh. Genesis 2:18-24 (NKJV)

It was not good that I withdrew into myself. I am not very good company to myself. I need others in my life. Withdrawal makes me sick. It only gives me my point of view, and I do not grow closer to God by just being by myself.

The Bible says:

… not forsaking the assembling of ourselves together, as is the manner of some, but exhorting one another, and so much the more as you see the Day approaching. Hebrews 10:25 (NKJV)

For you were once darkness, but now you are light in the Lord. Walk as children of light (for the fruit of the Spirit is in all goodness, righteousness, and truth), finding out what is acceptable to the Lord. And having no fellowship with the unfruitful works of darkness, but rather expose them. For it is shameful even to speak of those things which are done by them in secret. But all things that are exposed are made manifest by the light, for whatever makes manifest is light. Therefore He says: "Awake you who sleep, Arise from the dead, And Christ will give you light."

See then that you walk circumspectly, not as fools but as wise, redeeming the time, because the days are evil.

Therefore do not be unwise, but understand what the will of the Lord is. And do not be drunk with wine, in which is dissipation; but be filled with the Spirit, speaking to one another in psalms and hymns and spiritual songs, singing and making melody in your heart to the Lord, giving thanks always for all things to God the Father in the name of our Lord Jesus Christ, submitting to one another in the fear of God. Ephesians 5:8-21 (NKJV)

But the fruit of the Spirit is love, joy, peace, longsuffering, kindness, goodness, faithfulness, gentleness, self-control. Against such there is no law. Galatians 5:22-23 (NKJV)

I started talking to Bro. Randy and Pam, and now to Dr. Snowden and Dr. Wieck. I have tried to talk to God about my problems. But every time I start to remember, I slam the door shut again in my mind. I do not know why it is so hard for me to talk. Bro. Jim at church calls me Gabby. I think because I was so quiet. But I guess I have kind of grown into my nick-name. Anyway, everyone at church has encouraged me to talk. Except I could feel the depression getting worse. I asked a few of the ladies at the church to pray for me, and Cindy anointed me with oil and they laid hands on me and prayed for me. My concern is always - how much do I tell and how much do I not tell.

The ladies who prayed for me the Wednesday night that Cindy anointed me with oil taught me there is a difference between having an impure thought and it becoming a sin. It is not a sin to be tempted. It is a sin to give in to temptation and sin.

Turn at my rebuke; Surely I will pour out my spirit on you; I will make my words known to you. Because I have called and you refused, I have stretched out my hand and no one regarded, Because you disdained all my counsel, And would have none of my rebuke, I also will laugh at your calamity; I will mock when your terror comes, When your terror comes like a storm, And your destruction comes like a whirlwind, When distress and anguish come upon you. "Then they will call on me, but I will not answer; They will seek me diligently, but they will not find me. Because they hated knowledge And did not choose the fear of the LORD, They would have none of my counsel And despised my every rebuke. Therefore they shall eat the fruit of their own way, And be filled to the full with their own fancies. For the turning away of the simple will slay them, And the complacency of fools will destroy them; But whoever listens to me will dwell in safety, And will be secure, without fear of evil." Proverbs 1:23-33 (NKJV)

I have forsaken God. Therefore, God will not deliver me in times of distress. Idols take God's place. God will give me up to the lusts of my heart. God will give me up to dishonorable passions. If I do not acknowledge God —God will give me up. He did it with Samson and King Saul — I am no different. If I do not listen and obey when God calls, if I refuse to listen or heed, if I ignore God's counsel, if I do not change at His reproof — God will laugh at my calamity. God will mock when terror strikes me. When terror strikes me like a storm and my calamity comes like a whirlwind, when distress and anguish come upon me, then I will call upon God and He will not answer. I will seek Him but will not find Him.

I would have <u>lost heart</u>, unless I had believed That I would see the goodness of the LORD In the land of the living. Wait on the LORD; Be of good courage, And He shall strengthen your heart; Wait, I say, on the LORD. Psalm 27:13-14 (NKJV)

Therefore we do not lose heart. Even though our outward man is perishing, yet the inward man is being renewed day by day. For our light affliction, which is but for a moment, is working for us a far more exceeding and eternal weight of glory, while we do not look at the things which are seen, but at the things which are not seen. For the things which are seen are temporary, but the things which are not seen are eternal. 2 Corinthians 4:16-18 (NKJV)

Lost heart in *Webster's Encyclopedia Dictionary of the English Language* means despair, nothing lower, the end, depression, anxiety, sad words. Getting old is not much fun. Friends precede us in death. If the only thing I have to live for is this life—it is over. I would despair. But Jesus said I go to prepare a place for you. We are going to go to the land of the living. Eternal life begins the moment we get saved.

Jesus is speaking:

"Let not your heart be troubled; you believe in God, believe also in Me. In My Father's house are many mansions; if it were not so, I would have told you. I go to prepare a place for you. And If I go to prepare a place for you, I will come again and receive you to Myself; that where I am, there you may be also. And where I go you know and the way you know."

Thomas said to Him, "LORD, we do not know where You are going, and how can we know the way?"

Jesus said to him, "I am the way, the truth, and the life. No one comes to the Father, except through Me. "If you had known Me, you would have known My Father also; and from now on you know Him and have seen Him."
John 14:1-7 (NKJV)

People think I do not care, but I do. They think I am dumb, but I am not. They think I am silent, but I talk to God a lot.

From the Daily Devotional — "Our love is here to stay" by Tony Evans.

Dear Jesus, I relinquish control of my body to Your touch, Your care, Your caress and Your love, my Husband to be. In Jesus Name, Amen.

All that time I looked for another, Jesus was always there waiting for me. I tried other ways to be loved. I found Jesus to be the Lover of my soul. Jesus meets my needs, deep needs, needs no one else can touch. Jesus knows what it takes to love me. I found the fact that He never gave up on me to be what impressed me the most. Jesus never quit loving me even when I was very unloving back to Him; He forgave me each time I asked. Sometimes it was for the same sin repeated over and over again. Are you in a religion or are you in a relationship with Jesus? It is all about relationship with Jesus.

In the Hebrew culture, when the groom gets married, after the marriage is when he begins to court his new bride and helps her fall in love with him. Jesus has a whole eternity ahead to encourage us to fall in love with Him. I just know right now I am satisfied with His love like never before in my life. I had other loves in my life, but no one else even comes close to meeting my needs like Jesus can and does. As an added bonus to being married to Jesus—Abba, who will remain always as my DADDY will also become my Father-in-law one day when I get to heaven. I look forward to that blessing. Pa was a great example to me of what a Father-in-law should be. He taught me unconditional love.

Jesus said,

> *"And whenever you stand praying, if you have anything against anyone, forgive him, that your Father in heaven may also forgive you your trespasses. But if you do not forgive, neither will your Father in heaven forgive your trespasses."* Mark 11:25-26 (NKJV)

Just ask Him to show you His love and He will — over and over as many times as you can ask Him He can show you His love. Have you asked for anything? Ask God to show you His love. Look for an exceeding, abundant answer to your prayer because that is how Jesus answers.

> *Now to Him who is able to do exceedingly abundantly above all that we ask or think according to the power that works in us, to Him be glory in the church by Christ Jesus to all generations, forever and ever. Amen.* Ephesians 3:20-21 (NKJV)

Abba, let's start with thank You and I praise You. Thank You—I went and met Dr. Snowden for the first time today. I like him, he listens and talks with me and he asks questions. We talked for an hour and a half. Jen and her family took me to the appointment. I would never have come to the saving grace of God if these things had not happened in my life. I praise God for how You have formed me. You are truly the Potter and I am just the clay. All the other times, when I went though a manic episode, I have shut down and disconnected with God and quit talking, sometimes for months at a time. It was Dr. Snowden that noticed I would disconnect with God sometimes. We are working hard for that not to happen this time.

Abba, forgive me for lack of confidence in You, God. I trust You even when things do not seem to be in Your control. You are in control at all times. I have learned that from the Daniel Bible study I went to last year. It was a Beth Moore Bible study taught by Cindy. I also am learning You are in control from Bro. Randy's messages on the book of Daniel. God, You revealed Your plan hundreds of years before it happened, and You revealed Your plan even for the last days here on earth. Bro. Randy said we are in the feet and toes in the time frame of today. Nebuchadnezzar saw an image. The head was gold, and it represented the Babylonian empire. The chest and arms of the image were silver and represented the Medes and Persian empire who crushed the Babylonians. Then the torso and legs of the image were bronze and it represented Alexander the Great and the Greek empire. Four leaders replaced him, and then the Roman empire took over which was represented as feet and toes of iron mixed with clay of the image. We are near the end times.

Abba, You foretold it all just the way it happened. You are trustworthy. You have a perfect plan. Jesus, everything happened just like it had to in Your life. You were born to a virgin, KING of kings and LORD of lords. You were taken to Egypt to protect You as a little baby. As a child, You went to church (the temple) and spoke with the teachers and worshiped. You lived thirty-three years upon this earth to find out what it was like to be human and for us to learn what You are like. Jesus,

You died on the cross a cruel death for our sins, You never sinned. You arose from the dead on the third day just as it was prophesied. You ate and drank with the disciples and taught them what they needed to know. You went back to heaven. Then You sent Your Holy Spirit to be our Helper. And everything happened according to scriptures written hundreds of years before it happened. In the book of Revelation it says You, Jesus, are coming back for us, Your church. What a glorious day that will be! The book of Revelation and the book of Daniel in the Bible will be read like a newspaper as the things prophesied in the Bible start coming true for those who will be left behind.

Abba, You are in control. I praise You and I thank You. You are worthy of my love and relationship. I love You. If I do not place my faith and expectation in God, I end up just trusting in myself or someone else. That is a long way from the dependence I can have in Jesus, Abba, and the Holy Spirit.

Abba, Jesus, Holy Spirit, You are so worthy of my placing my faith in You. I expect You to do great things in my life. I am sorry for my sins when I have placed my faith in myself or others like Buh. Gladly I place my expectations and faith back in Christ, You, Abba, and Your Holy Spirit. Fill me with Your Holy Spirit. Fill me with Your love.

Things that happen may hurt. I may not understand Your ways, but I can trust You through it, You are so worthy of my praise and I praise You. Thank You that You are in control. I place my faith in You.

Abba, Please, give me victory over these dreams, so I do not dream them anymore. Forgive me for having them. I am sorry I even have to ask. I pray for the mind of Christ. Abba, prepare me for Jesus to be my husband. Prepare my heart and mind, even my subconscious mind, to love Jesus as my Husband, Savior and LORD. Forgive me; I turn from them to Christ. I repent and ask for Your help LORD God. Please, infiltrate even my dreams. Help me. In Jesus Name I place it in Your hands.

Abba, is depression a sin to me? I take my medicine as I should now, that means I take my medicine all of the time even when I am very level and not manic or depressed. If you were diabetic you would take your medicine every day even when you feel good. It is the same way with bipolar medicine. I see my doctors on a regular schedule. I try to do what they say. I have friends and family who care about me. And I know You love me. Forgive me—for so long I was "sin sick." I was not asking for forgiveness so I was sick. I try not to go too long before I ask You, God, what my sins are and confess them to You and ask for forgiveness. I want a relationship with You, Jesus. I need it. I crave it. There is a hole only You can fill in my life. Fill me with Your Holy Spirit. I pray for a sound mind. I pray for the mind of Christ.

Thank You that this manic depression will not last forever, not even in this lifetime. Sometimes I am depressed—sometimes I am manic—sometimes I am as normal as I can be. Is it a sin to be depressed or manic? I know when I bring it to You, God; You bring me out of it. You simply walk with me through it—back to a sound mind. But what about the times I am sick? I thank You also for the times when I am depressed, and I thank You for the times when I am manic. Most of all I thank You for saving me so when You take me home to Heaven to be with you permanently, I will be healed. I will know a joy that is so unspeakable it boggles my mind. I cannot even comprehend it. No words can explain it. Joy, true unhindered joy awaits us in Heaven. I give You my every heart beat. I choose to live for You. Until I go to heaven, I choose joy in the journey as I walk with You through trials, persecutions and the testing of my faith. May You find me full of faith in You, LORD. Thank You and I praise You for manic and depression. Thank You that there will not be a hint of it in heaven.

Abba, a few moments of honesty bring my sin quickly to mind. I see it. So do You. Let me see it in the same way You do—in all of its nastiness. I yield to You. I want a full understanding of the things that have kept my heart dry and at a distance from You. I see it all now—not just the "acceptable, on the surface" sins, but the ones I have hidden and nurtured for years. I go by how I feel and sometimes I feel rotten. And my moods reflect how I feel that day. It should not matter how I feel. Forgive me for my moodiness. The devil knows what buttons to push in me to get a reaction. Touchy and resentment go hand in hand. When I am criticized, I do not like it. My feelings get hurt, and I feel resentment.

Abba, forgive me for being touchy and resentful. Help me hear what You say to me and not go by feelings. Teach me to love always. Deliver me from the devil's hands. Build up a hedge around me to protect me from what he tries to do. I do not want to be blind to what he does in my life. Shine Your light God on his schemes. I pray for the power of Christ in me. I pray fill me with You Holy Spirit's love, joy, peace and faithfulness to trust You with all my days.

Thank You for bringing my sins to light. I cannot imagine my private life without this burden; but I am here, right now in faith, asking that You take it all away from me. No more covering. No more hiding. No more rationalizing. I believe that You are stirring a revival within me, and I know this dealing with sin has to come first. So I am coming in faith that You will help me, forgive me and help me know I am forgiven. I lose out of loving a lot of people when I do not care. I need to love them. Empower me to love them.

Abba, I ask for Your forgiveness. I want to be like You, God. I want to love like You—unconditionally. I want to care about people in my life, really care. Help me love all people like You, Abba. Fill me with Your Holy Spirit to love people. Fill me with Your Holy Spirit's gentleness, kindness, long suffering and self control. I am rude to people—I interrupt people talking instead of waiting for a time to speak. I do not want to be rude to anyone anymore. Forgive me.

Abba, I did not understand You, maybe I still do not. But You are close now-"closer than my very breath" as Bro. Jim says. You are in me. Dr. Snowden says it seems I disconnect from You, God. I never connected with You until I bent down on my knees at the trailer house in east Texas and You saved me. But I can tell when I disconnect with You now. I have tried every way possible not to disconnect with You this time. I kept talking with You and with the people You have placed in my life at this time that are my counselors and doctors. I have tried to stay connected to You through writing this book. I do not know if it will help anyone else, but it has been good for me to write it. I pray it will be good for others who read it.

Thank You that I am not afraid to go out of my room and the house. Thank You for Bro. Randy and Pam, Bro. Jim and Sandra, Bro. Jimmy and Cindy, Dr. Snowden, Dr. Wieck, Dr. Greer and Dr. Tom. Thank You for medicines that correct the chemical imbalance in my brain. Thank You for Tracie, Jodie, Andy and Crystal who just listen and talk with me. Thank You for Your Holy Spirit and that He takes my prayers and translates them into something You can listen to and act upon. Thank You for the privilege of prayer. Thank You for Jesus that He loves me so much that He died for me on the cross. I praise You and I thank You that three days later He rose from the dead and He walked and taught and ate and lived for 40 days on this earth afterwards before going back to heaven. Thank You, Jesus that You are preparing a place for us in heaven for eternity to take us to live with You forever. Thank You, Jesus, that You are coming back for Your church—all the believers who have trusted in Christ, Your Bride—the Church. Thank You Abba, my DADDY that You adopted me into Your family and newborn into Your Kingdom. Thank You for creating this world by speaking it into existence. Thank You for saving me. I pray others will come to know You in a close personal relationship. I praise You and I thank You for all things. Forgive me for withdrawing from You and disconnecting. Thank You, You never let me go. I praise You.

Abba, I have had impure thoughts. Please forgive me. Thank You there is victory over sin in Jesus. Impure thoughts lead to impure speech and impure speech leads to impure actions. I think a sin, then I speak a sin and then I do a sin and it could all happen in a split second. Thank You, I ask You to forgive me and cleanse me and make me whole again.

I wanted someone who did not belong to me. He is married and belongs to his wife. I told some of the ladies in our church, and they prayed for me that I would gain victory and not love someone I should not.

The worst consequence of my sin would be separation from You, God. I do not want that. I do not want any of this sin—I do not want the thoughts. I want it stopped now. I turn from my sin now. The best I know how; now, I turn from my sin. I do not want it to go any further in my thoughts. I do not want it to ever even become an action or a voice. I do not want anything to do with this sin. Forgive me of thinking what I have been thinking. I pray for victory in Christ. Jesus is my Husband-to-be. Thank You for forgiving me. Thank You that You have listened to me. When there were few I could go to about this sin, You listened and guided me to wise counsel on this earth and in Heaven above and in Your Word the Bible. Thank You and I praise You now for Your forgiveness, Your counsel, and Your love that would not let me go to another. I belong to Jesus. I am His and He is mine. I pray for strength. I pray to stay this course back to You, Jesus. Help me to understand forgiveness. Help me forgive like You forgive. Help me love without eros (error love). Help me repent.

Abba, I simply ask You to forgive me. He does not belong to me. Enough said. Forgive me. I turn back to You, Jesus. Abba, You know my heart. I love Jesus, but You also know my past record and this sin besets me. Continue to help me. I pray for victory in Jesus.

Abba, if I hate Your knowledge God and do not choose to fear You LORD and not have any of Your counsel and despise all of Your reproof—I shall eat the fruit of my ways and have my fill of my own devises. God, You will say, "Carol is joined with an idol; leave her alone." Those are the words I fear the most. "Leave her alone." Please forgive me. My idol is the created not You the Creator. I am sorry I have grown so far away from You. We are distanced. I will do whatever You ask; whatever it takes to get back to You. I just do not understand turning away from my sin. How? How do I do that? Is it a choice? Is it Your surgery? All I know is I do not want to be alone without You. I turn from my sin.

Can You do some watering and cultivating and pulling some sin weeds in my life? Can You teach me how to do these things too? I need a downpour of revival, in my soul and over my life. I need 1,000 refinements at once. Turn up the heat in my life and skim off the dross of sin in my life. My sins—I own up to them. Forgive me.

Abba, I cherish my time with You. God, it is very special. And You show me what I look like now to You. I do not want anything interfering with my relationship with You. No sin is worth that. You love me, You cannot love me anymore, and You cannot love me any less. You love me and You show that love to me by meeting needs deep down inside of me, such as just having someone to talk to—You, God talk to me. Thank You that amazes me. I am in awe that the God of the universe talks and listens and communicates with me. Abba, You started with one word. You spoke my name and You continue to speak to me in different ways by different people and from Your Word the Bible. You confirm in my heart what You want me to do, or say, or how to act and react. No sin is worth losing You, no sin. Please forgive me. Thank You Abba that You forgive sin and that it is not permanent unless we never ask for forgiveness in the first place.

Abba, forgive me for being so quiet. I have a message to tell. Am I telling anyone Jesus is the answer to any problem we have? He is the answer, no ifs, ands or buts about it. If you need anything, you can find the solution is Jesus every time. No one can solve problems faster than You, Jesus. I ask in Jesus Name and to His glory, Amen.

(35)

Sin = Separation from God

*I*t does not matter what the sin is. Sin separates us from God. There are a lot of other consequences to this sin, but not being in relationship with God is reason enough not to sin.

From the *Webster's Encyclopedic Dictionary of the English language*

Purge means:

> To cleanse, purify, clean from impurities or contamination, physical or spiritual:
> Purge me with hyssop and I shall be clean
> (law) To clear oneself of an accusation, charge, or suspicions; to wipe out, expiates an offense by suffering punishment:
> The defendant has already purged his offense, in other words: by undergoing punishment
>
> *Purge me with hyssop, and I shall be clean; Wash me, and I shall be whiter than snow. Make me hear joy and gladness That the bones You have broken may rejoice. Hide Your face from my sins, And blot out all my iniquities. Create in me a clean heart, O God, And renew a*

steadfast spirit within me. Do not cast me away from Your presence, And do not take Your Holy Spirit from me. Restore to me the joy of Your salvation, And uphold me by Your generous Spirit. Then I will teach transgressors Your ways, And sinners shall be converted to You. Deliver me from the guilt of bloodshed, O God, The God of my salvation, And my tongue shall sing aloud of Your righteousness. O Lord, open my lips, And my mouth shall show forth Your praise. For You do not desire sacrifice, or else I would give it; You do not delight in burnt offering. The sacrifices of God are a broken spirit, A broken and a contrite heart—These, O God, You will not despise. Psalm 51:7-17 (NKJV)

Abba, this is my prayer to You. Please forgive me. I am guilty. It was my sin that killed Jesus. I am so sorry He had to die to do it, but thank You so much that He died to save us from our sin. And if I had been the only one who had ever become a Christian, Jesus still would have died for me. Thank You, Jesus died for all if they will only choose Him to be their Savior. Thank You does not seem enough, but that is what You ask. Thank You, Thank You, Thank You, forever Thank You. I praise You, God. In Jesus Name, Amen.

August Saturday PM 8-23-08

While we look not at the things which are seen, but at the things not seen: for the things which are seen are temporal; but the things which are not seen are eternal. 2 Corinthians 4:18(KJV)

Then Jesus said to those Jews who believed Him, "If you abide in My word, you are My disciples indeed. And you shall know the truth, and the truth shall make you free. John 8:31-32 (NKJV)

Abba, thank You there is victory in Jesus. The "man" is back to being my brother in Christ. Thank You for Your power through the blood of Jesus over sin in my life. I love You, LORD Jesus with all my heart, and soul, and mind and strength. Thank You and I praise You and I praise You and I praise You! Thank You for the ladies who prayed specifically for me about this sin in my life. Thank You that You listen and answer prayer. I love "him" with agape love now and not eros (in error love). Thank You, for Your Trinity God, thank You to all three of You, Father, Jesus and Holy Spirit. I praise You for victory over sin. Control me by Your Spirit. My destiny is Jesus.

Thank You, Abba, for forgiving me and bringing me through this to the other side. Thank You for the ladies who prayed with me and supported me. Thank You and I praise You for Your agape love. You love us and You are not in it for the sex. You love us because You can and God, You are so good at it. God with us is the meaning of Immanuel, God with us. God is with me, so I do not have to long for another. Jesus is enough. Thank You.

Abba, I fear You. It is a healthy fear. It is a reverence for God. I have a respect of You, LORD. It is an awe of who You are, LORD. And yet You did not squish me like a bug. You did not quit loving me. You forgave me. I thought I had to ask one sin by one sin to be forgiven and if I missed one I was out of grace. But Jesus' blood covers our sins, every sin completely—past, present and future sins. I do not know why; I just did not get this truth until Saturday night August 16, 2008 I just did not get this truth. But God, I do now!

I praise You God. You got through to me; get it through to others too. It is not works although we are to serve, not gifts though we are to give, not feelings because feelings are temporal; they change all the time. If I go by feelings, they are temporary. When I am going through it at the time, it is not fun, and I do not want to feel this way. If I go by feelings, I may not feel saved. Being saved is a fact, not a feeling. Help us to know this truth and this truth shall set us free.

Abba, I want joy. That is what we are striving for with Dr. Snowden in our counseling sessions—Joy. It is all grace, unmerited, undeserved and much of the time at least in my life unasked for grace. It is all God. And our response should be gratitude, so let's start there.

Thank You for saving me. Unworthy that I am and I still sin against You. A lot of the time I do not understand You and Your ways, but I know now that I am forgiven completely and forever forgiven. I may fall down and sin, but You never have let me fall any further than my knees or to my face before You in repentance. God, You are good. You are the definition of the word good. God, You define love too. You loved us so much You sent Your only begotten Son, the love of Your life to this earth to die for us. Thank You and I praise You. Jesus never sinned, not one single time. Jesus came so we can be the love of His life too.

Abba, thank You for forgiving me of all my past sins, present sins, and future sins. That was something I did not understand until I listened to Bro. Randy preach on the CD of the morning sermon of 8-10-08, he said something like, that he had been saying it since he had started preaching at our church a year ago. Only I did not take note of it until I realized when You, God, repeat something I better listen. So I replayed the CD and really listened. I listened and believed: Jesus paid for my sins—past, present and future. You make me justified—just as if I had never sinned. So much of the book of Ephesians did not get through my brain. But God! I get it! Thank You Jesus for forgiving me by paying the price for my sin by dying on the cross and paying the sin penalty for my sin. I praise You God. Thank You, Jesus. Paid in full is written all over these pages describing my sins. Not guilty is shouted over me. I praise You

God, I praise You. I praise You! Praise God, Abba, and thank You for giving up Jesus for a time. Thank You, Jesus, for volunteering to come to earth and die for me. Thank You that it was not just for me but for anyone else who will accept Jesus' death as full payment for their sins. Thank You for loving me.

Thank You for Your grace, mercy, loving kindnesses and tender intimacies. Father, forgive me for being so stubborn; help me to do things Your way and in Your timing. I was stubborn about this homework assignment. I had a lot of sins marked in the book *Downpour*. I have stubbornly procrastinated against finishing this assignment. I firmly plant my feet when I am stubborn. People cannot change my mind even if they try. I fight against You, instead of on Your side, I fight against You. Time does not always heal all wounds, but I have to bring my sins and my wounds to You, God, so You can forgive me and heal me. The sooner I do that the better.

Abba, Forgive me for being so stubborn. I yield to Your Holy Spirit. Change me, O God. Transform me, When Jay was a little boy, he liked to play with toys called Transformers. My grandchildren Garrett and Colby love to play with Transformers; they will sit for hours changing the toys back and forth over and over again. I need You to change me—transform me to be like Christ. I do not want to transform back to the old way I was. Thank You and I praise You Abba. Help me obey You. Help me do what You tell me to do when You tell me to do it. Help me finish this homework of dealing with and asking forgiveness for my sins. Thank You and I praise You. In Jesus Name, Amen.

(36)

Heaven and Hell

I never opened up to anyone until I went to a revival meeting where Don Piper was speaking of heaven. I stayed that night after the revival was over, at the pastor's invitation, and when everyone was gone, I got to talk with Don Piper. I only told him of one thing. My story is so different from his - he saw heaven - I heard hell. One day they sent me to another building of the state hospital to be tested. While I was sitting and waiting out in the hall I heard a creaking sound and then a scream. It happened over and over again. Screams worse than any the movies can produce. Over and over and over and over again I heard screams, awful blood curdling screams, each one a different person's. Each scream would be loud at first and then gradually to quietness as if they were going down into a bottomless pit. It reminded me of a person's entrance to hell. People scream as they realize they are entering hell. Satan plays for keeps, but he is not going to let you scream forever, he is not going to listen to you scream. The Bible says it will be weeping and gnashing of teeth forever and ever and ever.

Jesus wants to hear from you. You do not have to scream. He can hear your thoughts and prayers. You do not even have to voice them out loud. Pray in your heart to God that hears. Tell Him you need Him and want Him to save you. Give Him your heart and soul. Repent of your sins that means you do not do them anymore with God's help. You ask and pray "in Jesus Name, Amen."

I want people to know now how to be saved. The first few seconds of the people's entrance into hell is what I heard. Darkness and the aloneness of hell is what I felt. I have been afraid to talk until now.

The first second of Hell there will be a feeling of lostness, beyond help, beyond being forgiven, beyond hope of ever being saved, that feeling will last forever and it will be too late to do anything about it.

You are still alive, so you can make that choice right now to choose Jesus as your Savior and LORD. Do you believe in heaven and hell? It does not matter if you believe or not, you will spend eternity in one of those two places when you die—depending on if you trust Jesus to save you now or not, while you are still on this earth. Are you afraid of God? He will forgive you if you ask. He will become your Abba DADDY, your Heavenly Father.

What is sin to me? Sin separates me from God. Sin is doing anything I want to do instead of what God wants me to do. Sin is death—spiritual death instantly which eventually leads to physical death. Without Jesus sin leads to a living death in hell for eternity—forever in hunger, thirst, fire, brimstone, darkness and torment.

> *But the sons of the kingdom will be cast out into outer darkness. There will be weeping and gnashing of teeth."* Matthew 8:12 (NKJV)

Weeping and gnashing of teeth that is what hell will be like.
With no end.
No more time.
Just forever.
And no way out once you get there.

Have you ever been hungry where your stomach growled or that empty feeling became a burning feeling in your stomach? In hell there is eternal hunger. In hell there is eternal thirst. Not one morsel of food, not one drop of water for the rest of eternity. Hell is never ending—always hungry and always longing for water, your mouth so dry you cannot swallow or talk—forever in torment.

Choose Jesus now. There will be no second chance after you go to hell. You will not be alone. Satan and the demons will be locked in hell with you. They fight dirty. They lie. They do not pull any punches. Evil is what they are and evil is what they do. And they are going to be angry and furious at anyone there in hell with them. Would you be afraid? Would you be afraid to be touched because it could be the devil or his demons? Weeping and gnashing of teeth, that is what the Bible says it will be. It is repeated seven times in the Bible when God repeats Himself you better listen.

The Son of Man will send out His angels, and they will gather out of His kingdom all things that offend, and those who practice lawlessness, and will cast them into the furnace of fire. There will be wailing and gnashing of teeth. Then the righteous will shine forth as the sun in the kingdom of their Father. He who has ears to hear, let him hear! Matthew 13:41-43 (NKJV)

"Again, the kingdom of heaven is like a dragnet that was cast into the sea and gathered some of every kind, which, when it was full, they drew to shore; and they sat down and gathered the good into vessels, but threw the bad away. So it will be at the end of the age. The angels will come forth, separate the wicked from among the just, and cast them into the furnace of fire. There will be wailing and gnashing of teeth." Jesus said to them, *"Have you understood all these things?"* Matthew 13:47-51 (NKJV)

And Jesus answered and spoke to them again by parables and said: "The kingdom of heaven is like a certain king who arranged a marriage for his son, and sent out his servants to call those who were invited to the wedding; and they were not willing to come. Again, he sent out other servants, saying, 'Tell those who are invited, "See, I have prepared my dinner; my oxen and fatted cattle are killed, and all things are ready. Come to the wedding." 'But they made light of it and went their ways, one to his own farm, another to his business. And the rest seized his servants, treated them spitefully, and killed them. But when the king heard about it, he was furious. And he sent out his armies, destroyed those murderers, and burned up their city. Then he said to his servants, 'The wedding is ready, but those who were invited were not worthy. Therefore go into the highways, and as many as you find, invite to the wedding.' So those servants went out into the highways and gathered together all whom they found, both bad and good. And the wedding hall was filled with guests. But when the king came in to see the guests, he saw a man there who did not have on a wedding garment. So he said to him, 'Friend, how did you come in here without a wedding garment?' And he was speechless. Then the king said to the servants, 'Bind him hand and foot, take him away, and cast him into outer darkness; there will be weeping and gnashing of teeth. "For many are called, but few are chosen'. Matthew 22:1-14 (NKJV)

Jesus is speaking:

"Who then is a faithful and wise servant, whom his master made ruler over his household, to give them food in due season? Blessed is that servant whom his master, when he comes, will find so doing. Assuredly, I say to you that he will make him ruler over all his goods. But if that evil servant says in his heart, 'My

master is delaying his coming,' and begins to beat his fellow servants, and to eat and drink with the drunkards. The master of that servant will come on a day when he is not looking for him and at an hour that he is not aware of, and will cut him in two and appoint him his portion with the hypocrites. There shall be weeping and gnashing of teeth. Matthew 24:45-51 (NKJV)

Jesus is *speaking:*

"For the kingdom of heaven is like a man traveling to a far country who called his own servants and delivered his goods to them. And to one he gave five talents, to another two, and to another one, to each according to his own ability; and immediately he went on a journey. Then he who had received the five talents went and traded with them, and made another five talents. And likewise he who had received two gained two more also. But he who had received one went and dug in the ground, and hid his lord's money. After a long time the lord of these servants came and settled accounts with them.

So he who had received five talents came and brought five other talents, saying, 'Lord, you delivered to me five talents; look, I have gained five more talents besides them.' His lord said to him, 'Well done, good and faithful servant; you were faithful over a few things, I will make you ruler over many things. Enter into the joy of your lord.' He also who had received two talents came and said, 'Lord, you delivered to me two talents; look, I have gained two more talents besides them.' His lord said to him, 'Well done, good and faithful servant; you have been faithful over a few things, I will make you ruler over many things. Enter into the joy of your lord.'

"Then he who had received the one talent came and said, 'Lord, I knew you to be a hard man, reaping where you have not sown, and gathering where you have not scattered seed. And I was afraid, and went and hid your talent in the ground. Look, there you have what is yours.'

"But his lord answered and said to him, 'You wicked and lazy servant, you knew that I reap where I have not sown, and gather where I have not scattered seed. So you ought to have deposited my money with the bankers, and at my coming I would have received back my own with interest. So take the talent from him, and give it to him who has ten talents.

'For to everyone who has, more will be given, and he will have abundance; but from him who does not have, even what he has will be taken away. And cast the unprofitable servant into the outer darkness. There will be weeping and gnashing of teeth.' Matthew 25:14-30 (NKJV)

Jesus is speaking:

And He went through the cities and villages, teaching, and journeying toward Jerusalem. Then one said to Him, "Lord, are there few who are saved?" And He said to them, "Strive to enter through the narrow gate, for many, I say to you, will seek to enter and will not be able. When once the Master of the house has risen up and shut the door, and you begin to stand outside and knock at the door, saying, 'Lord, Lord open for us,' and He will answer and say to you, 'I do not know you, where you are from, ' then you will begin to say, 'We ate and drank in Your presence, and You taught in our streets.' But He will say, 'I tell you I do not know you, where you are from. Depart from Me, all you workers of iniquity.'

There will be weeping and gnashing of teeth, when you see Abraham and Isaac and Jacob and all the prophets in the kingdom of God and yourselves thrust out. They will come from the east and the west, from the north and the south, and sit down in the kingdom of God. And indeed there are last who will be first, and there will be first who will be last." Luke 13:22-30 (NKJV)

Jesus does not want you to go to hell, hell was created for the devil and the demons. But that is where you will go if you are not saved.

The Lord is not slack concerning His promise, as some count slackness, but is longsuffering toward us, not willing that any should perish but that all should come to repentance. 2 Peter 3:9 (NKJV)

Jesus is the only way to not go to hell in the first place. Jesus died and paid the sin penalty for your sins so you would not have to. Trust Jesus and gain heaven. It is based on your decision you make right now while you are still alive. It cannot wait another minute. Your decision right now will have an eternal difference. This very moment could change your eternal destiny. Choose Jesus and you go to heaven instead of hell. That is a fact you trust by faith, and God gives us the faith to believe in His Son, Jesus. It is all grace. We do not earn it by doing good things. There are a lot of good people in hell right now because they would not accept Jesus as their Savior. If I could choose Jesus for you, I would, but I cannot, it has to be your decision. God will forgive you because Jesus paid the price for your sin when He suffered and died on the cross. Three days later He arose from the grave to prove His love for us.

Eternal death or eternal life?

The decision should be a no brainer. You should not have to even think on it. Choose life forever with Jesus by trusting in Jesus to save you. It is a personal decision; no one else can make it for you. Once you have accepted Jesus' salvation for yourself, He will never leave you nor forsake you. And you will be allowed to go to heaven. There is a pearly gate. But it only has a small entrance, only big enough for one person to go through it at a time. That is how Don Piper explained it at a revival when I went to hear him. Don Piper died for 90 minutes and came back to earth; while he was dead, his spirit went to the gate of heaven. He tells about it in his book *90 minutes in Heaven*. He talked about the magnitude of joy in Heaven. He told about a 1,000 songs being sung all at once in praise to God, but it sounding harmonious and not discord at all. He talked about all his family and the people who were instrumental in leading him to the LORD being outside the gate. Go through the door when you get to heaven. I want to see Jesus. I want to get through that entrance of the pearly gate and meet Jesus and God the Father and the Holy Spirit face to face.

Absent from the body is present with the LORD, that is what the Bible says,

> *So we are always confident, knowing that while we are at home in the body we are absent from the Lord. For we walk by faith, not by sight. We are confident, yes, well pleased rather to be absent from the body and to be present with the Lord.* 2 Corinthians 5:6-8 (NKJV)

In heaven there will be no more sickness and death. There is not that same assurance if your place is assigned to hell. Please do not chance torment forever in eternal fire.

Jesus died for all. But, not all will go to heaven. Only those who trust Jesus as their Savior and LORD will go to heaven. Jesus is the only way, there will never be another.

Jesus said to him, "I am the way, the truth, and the life. No one comes to the Father except through Me. John 14:6 (NKJV)

Choose Jesus. Heaven is for believers in Christ only. Believe in Jesus. You will never be sorry you did. No regrets, God works all things to our good. William Borden said it so well: "No reserves, No retreats, No regrets."

November (Saturday) 11-8-08

Eternity is a long time, but how do we get a grasp on how long eternity really is? The following is based on Bro. Kenneth's illustration he used in a sermon I heard as a child.

If a bird came and picked up one grain of sand every billion years and put it in a pile. By the time he picked up every grain of sand on the whole earth and on the ocean floor, it would not even have used a fraction of a billi-second of eternity's time. But picture this, the bird comes back and picks up one grain of sand again, every billion years. The bird could do this forever and it would still be just a billi-second of eternity's time. You will be in one of two places—Heaven or Hell. To get into Heaven you have to trust Jesus to save you while you are still on this earth. If you do not trust Jesus, Abba God has no choice but to send you to an eternity in Hell.

In heaven there is pure, indescribable joy, healing, love beyond measure and the light and presence of Jesus forever more. In hell: there is there is fire, darkness, depression, sadness, grief, suffering, pain, unquenchable thirst and hunger, and separation from God and the people He saves.

Choose wisely, eternity is forever. The decision has to be made now while you are still alive. Choose Jesus to gain a living eternity in Heaven that begins the moment you accept Him into Your heart and life. If you do not, you will live a living eternity in fire and brimstone in the place God made for the devil and his demons.

New life in Christ may cost you some friendships, but you gain more. Family members may not believe with you, but you gain the family of God. Jesus is worth any cost.

People do not understand why people have to die. When Jesus was in the garden before His crucifixion He prayed that night for us to see His glory. He died on the cross and three days later He arose. The disciples saw Him, He taught them 40 days then He went back to Heaven. Jesus wants us to see His glory. People die one by one and if they are saved they go to heaven. They see His glory; our objective is to go to see Jesus in all His glory. It is not a bad thing to die. Our last breath on earth is our first breath in Heaven, forever never thirsty, forever never hungry, forever never bored, forever never lonely, forever never sick, or maimed, or paralyzed, or blind, or deaf, forever with our loved ones, forever with Jesus and God the Father and the Holy Spirit. Forever glory in Heaven. Do not be afraid to die if you are saved. But if you are not saved you will go to hell, fire and torment forever. It does not matter if you believe in Hell or not. That is where you will go. Please trust Jesus now, before it is too late. There is no get out of hell free card. God does not play games. Jesus is the only way to be saved. You cannot be good enough to get out of going to hell. One sin is all it takes to send you there. Have you ever sinned? Then you need Jesus. Lying is a sin. Stealing is a sin. Adultery is a sin and Jesus put it on a level that if you just look at another in lust you are as guilty as if you did the act. Murder is a sin. Not believing in Jesus is a sin.

I learned this in Glorietta.
Spell sin: SIN

Notice there is an "I" in the middle of SIN. SIN is doing anything I want to do instead of what God wants me to do.
Simple Salvation

for all have sinned and fall short of the glory of God,
Romans 3:23 (NKJV)

We all sin even after becoming Christians, but we can ask God's forgiveness and His help to overcome the sins in our lives.

For the wages of sin is death, but the gift of God is eternal life in Christ Jesus our Lord. Romans 6:23 (NKJV)

It is an eternal living Hell if you do not trust Jesus as your Savior. You will want death to end it, but it will not. Forever you will want to die, but it is a living Hell, always wanting to die and never being able to get away from the torment and pain.

But God demonstrates His own love toward us, in that while we were still sinners, Christ died for us. Romans 5:8 (NKJV)

Jesus loved you to death. He died to pay for your sins on the cross. Jesus never sinned, so He was the perfect sacrifice for your sins that God accepts as payment for your sins if you will only trust Jesus as your Savior and LORD of your life.

that if you confess with your mouth the Lord Jesus and believe in your heart that God has raised Him from the dead, you will be saved. For with the heart one believes unto righteousness, and with the mouth confession is made unto salvation. Romans 10:9-10 (NKJV)

As soon as you stop and pray and ask Jesus to save you, you need to tell someone what just happened in your heart and life. Someone who has been praying for you to be saved needs to hear what just happened from your own mouth so they can rejoice with you that you just got saved and what Jesus just did in your life. Who is that person you can tell? Keep telling your story, lots of people need to hear it.

He came to His own, and His own did not receive Him. But as many as received Him, to them He gave the right to become children of God, to those who believe in His name: who were born, not of blood, nor the will of the flesh, nor of the will of man, but of God. John 1:11-13 (NKJV)

It is a birthing process. You were born into this world, and you are born into the kingdom of God by asking to be saved.

Jesus said to him, "I am the way, the truth, and the life. No one comes to the Father except through Me. "If you had known Me, you would have known My Father also; and from now on you know Him and have seen Him." John 14:6-7 (NKJV)

When you get Jesus, you get His Father too. You can call Him, Abba, too. Abba means He's a DADDY. He wants to be Your Heavenly DADDY too, and you get the Holy Spirit also.

And he brought them out and said, "Sirs, what must I do to be saved?" So they said, "Believe on the Lord Jesus Christ, and you will be saved, you and your household." Acts 16:30-31 (NKJV)

God gives you the faith to believe. If you do not believe right now, at least ask God to help you believe. He will help you. God loves you into the kingdom. God is good all the time; all the time God is good.

Jesus died on the cross for my sin and your sin. Jesus did not stay dead. Three days later He arose from the dead. Jesus is alive and He wants to be alive in you. Trust God. Say this prayer out loud to God who hears and will help you.

Abba, I am a sinner. I want You to forgive me of my sins. I want to believe that Jesus died on the cross for my sin. Help me with my unbelief. Father, this is true, will You help me believe. I give Jesus my life. In Jesus Name, Amen.

It is all true.

Now tell someone your story, it is your testimony of how Jesus just saved you!

Jesus spoke in the Bible 365 times in different ways by different people: Do not fear. I fear God. I respect God. I am in awe of God. I revere God, but if a person does not trust Jesus as LORD and Savior now — God's only choice for them is to go to hell forever. There is no way out once you get there. People need to know now. But are we getting the word out that there is a Savior in Jesus Christ? Are we really even trying? Are we using every means available? Are we praying for those who do go and tell about Jesus? Are we giving till it hurts? Are we going, maybe not across the world but maybe even just next door to a neighbor? I am talking to me too when I ask these questions. What am I doing to get the message of Jesus saving power to a lost world or maybe just one person who needs to hear my story? Hell is real. Satan is real, and he fights dirty! Take the d away from devil and you end up with evil and that is what the devil is. Satan hates us because he hates Jesus!

But this is what was spoken by the prophet Joel:

> *"And it shall come to pass afterward That I will pour out of My Spirit on all flesh; Your sons and daughters shall prophesy, Your old men shall dream dreams. Your young men shall see visions, And also on My menservants and on My maidservants I will pour out My Spirit in those days. "And I will show wonders in the heavens and in the earth: Blood and fire and pillars of smoke. The sun shall be turned into darkness, And the moon into blood, Before the coming of the great and awesome day of the LORD. And it shall come to pass That whoever calls on the name of the LORD Shall be saved. Joel 2:28-32 (NKJV)*

God, it was darkness before You got a hold of my life of disease, sickness and sin. I was empty — now You fill me, heal me and shine Your light in me and out through me. I was sad before, now I have Your joy, and I know You are restoring me to a right Spirit with You. Someday in heaven I will be complete. Until then keep working on me. Do not ever let me go. I do not ever want to go back to my old life. Change me, transform me, and help me bloom where You plant me. Shine, Jesus, shine through the cracks in me that You have left on purpose. Let Your Holy Spirit bubble out through those cracks and over the top. Fill me with Your Holy Spirit to overflowing.

Abba, I love You. How do You want to be loved? Thank You for loving me, help me love You in return. Help me love those I can see until I am with You whom I cannot see right now. Help me love people who are hard to love. Help me love people who will never love me in return. Help me to be color blind until I do not notice the differences but only notice how we are alike. I am not easy to love, but You love me anyway. I pray for grace upon grace so I can give grace away to other people. Help me care about other people all over the world. But let me start with the people with whom I come into contact daily. Teach me as I go how to make an impact on Your world, changing lives one at a time. Help me be satisfied with Your timing in saving people. That may never be 1,000s at a time. Help me be satisfied with the one at a time You save. Please confuse, confound and dismay the devil and the demons. I pray they will be so disappointed with how few there will be left behind when You, Jesus, come back to get Your Bride, the church. The rapture will happen, until then pour out Your Holy Spirit on us and fill us. You said in the last days You would pour out Your Holy Spirit on us. Fill us and lead us to those who need Jesus. I want others to fall madly in love with You, too. Help us share Jesus with people who do not know You yet. Help us to love You enough to want to share You with other people who are lost. I do not want anyone to go to hell because they have never heard about Jesus. But if they do not believe in You, Jesus, God has no other choice but to send them there. I ask in the Blessed Name of my Jesus, Amen.

(37)

LORD Bring a
Downpour in my Life!

I need You, Jesus, I need You Abba Father, I need You Holy Spirit. I desperately need to know all three of You have been in my life during the good and the bad. I need to know whether You want me to remember or forget what has happened in the past. I need a future with You. I need to love You with all my heart and soul and mind and strength. I need You to love me. Thank You and I praise You that You love me. I have to know and understand Jesus is God's will for me and that the definition of me is Jesus. I need my heart to belong only and always to Jesus. I need a DADDY, my Abba Father. I need a Savior, a Best Friend and a Big Brother and a Husband to be, my Jesus. I need a Helper, a Counselor and a Comforter, Holy Spirit. I need more of You.

Result: I am dependent on You, God every moment of the day. I need You. I need victory over my addiction to sin. I am prone to wander. Tie me to the horns of the altar. Center me on the altar. Drag me back if I even start to wander away. I plead the blood of Jesus upon my sins. Forgive me. I cannot right myself. I need You to pick me up and put me back on my feet. Jesus, show up and be God in me. You are my advocate. I need you to meet needs in me the right way—God's way. I ask in the Blessed Name above all names, the Name of Jesus, Amen.

October 1, 2003

Bro. Jonathan Hewitt came to preach revival services. I listened. God was talking to me. Jesus died for me—Jesus laid down His life for me. Bro. Jonathan said Jesus laid down on that cross voluntarily; no one had to force Him to get on that cross. He chose to be there for you and me because we needed Him. It was Jesus' love for us that held Him on the cross. The Israelites were God's chosen people, when they chose to reject their Savior, Jesus Christ; God opened His arms to us Gentiles. Gentiles are anyone who is not an Israelite or the Jews as they are called today. That includes me, does it include you? God was talking to me the night of the revival when Jonathan Hewitt came to our church. At the time of invitation I went down to the front and took Bro. Ricky's hand and said four words, "I believe in Jesus." It was just four simple words that I meant with all my heart. That was a turning point in my life. I believed in Jesus instead of just about Jesus. From that moment on I believed it all. The Bible was not just a bunch of stories anymore. The Bible came alive—Jesus walks and talks and teaches me the pages. Jesus walks with me through my day and talks to me about personal things, little things that do not matter to anybody else but me and Him. Every word of the scripture is true, cover to cover. Discover for yourself what it says. Maybe start with the book of John. Read it, say it out loud, and write scriptures that speak to you and your problems. Pray back the scriptures to God as prayers. Memorize your favorites and the ones you do not want to forget. Meditate on what God says. Teach God's Word to someone else. Write down your prayers in a journal to see how God answers your prayers, that way you can keep track of God's activity in your life. In your journal write down scriptures you want to remember. God says to remember the things He does in our lives. "Count your blessings; name them one by one and it will surprise you what the LORD has done." God is with us. Ask Him to show you His love for you. He never tires of showing us He loves us. Write it down so you will not forget to say thank you to God for what He does in your life.

I did not believe for a long time. I sang Christian songs, I went to church as a child and teen, but I did not trust the Bible. I did not belong at church. Unbelief robbed me of precious years I could have been with my Savior, Jesus. My regret is that it took me so long to trust Him. Jesus completes me. He finishes me. Jesus is always with me. He is who my heart has always longed for all my life. Jesus is my Savior, my King of kings and LORD of lords, my Big Brother, my Husband to be and my Best Friend. He is my destiny.

Thank You, Jesus, You died on the cross for me, in my place. It should have been me, I deserved it, and You did not deserve it. Thank You and I praise You; You died in my place and You live in me. Thank You, You just kept on teaching me truth upon truth of Your scriptures in the Bible until believing You was a "no-brainer." I would have been a fool not to believe. It is easier to believe in Jesus than not to believe in Jesus. I pray that will be true in the lives of the people who read this book and Your Word the Bible. Savior, please save people now that is what Hosanna means. I ask in Jesus' Precious Name, Amen.

(38)

God Spoke!

Someone told me I do not let anyone else talk. So, I am silent again, except on these pages today. God quietly asked me this morning to be silent. Over and over again He asked me to be silent, a fast of silence. I am talking on these pages alone.

Am I well? I do not know. Someday I may have to go back in the hospital. I take my medications all the time, even when I feel good. I talk to my doctors. I am more whole, more at peace, more full of love and full of more joy than at any time in my whole entire life. And it is not manic. It is contentment with my Abba Father. Abba means He is a DADDY, my DADDY. It is a satisfaction with my Heavenly Father who loves me and wants His best for me. He wants that for you, too. Trust in Jesus, God, who gave His life for you and me. Ask Jesus Christ to be your Savior, too. But do not stop there. Every day you can have more of a relationship with Jesus, and God the Father, as your DADDY and the Holy Spirit too.

Abba, is this book just for me and my healing? Can it help anyone else? People are going through manic and depression right now. Could it help them? Would You speak to the people in church to help them understand better about mental illness and about You at the same time? I pray people will be helped by this book and saved by You at the same time.

Abba, thank You, for a day of silence. I pray You have heard the prayers of people being born into Your kingdom today and if not today, very, very soon. I praise You, God; I give all the glory to You. Thank You, while I was silent today, You gave me the scriptures for this book. I praise You.

Abba Father, I thank You God for You. I praise You that there are three persons in the God head. I praise You that You will never die again. I praise You that Jesus Christ will never have to pay the sin penalty ever again—that it was once and for all and it is finished. I praise You that Jesus is alive. I praise You for Your Holy Spirit, alive in us, alive forever more.

Abba, I praise You and I thank You. Life happens at a much faster pace now that I am a Christian. Life was so slow with long days and longer nights before I became a Christian. I tried to sleep my life away, a lot out of boredom and a lot out of depression.

I do not want my going to see Dr. Snowden to take the place of Your Holy Spirit! Your Holy Spirit has been my counselor now for years. And He is the best. He taught me and sold me on Jesus.

Why do I have to talk about it? And how much do I tell? Nothing is off limits with You. What about with Dr. Snowden? What do I say and stop me before I say too much. Put a watch guard on my mouth. But prompt me if I do not say enough. Help me remember. God, open doors of my memory that I have slammed close. Things I do not dare even to think about anymore. But above all Thy will, not my will be done. Why do I have to do this now and not when I get to Heaven? Dr. Snowden's words at the door when I left was "Let's try and get some joy back in your life."

I choose joy. It has been appropriated to me, and I choose joy. That is what Beth Moore taught me. I am choosing joy, and if it takes some work to get there, then I am rolling up my sleeves and I am ready to work at it. I just do not want to do it alone without You, Holy Spirit. I need You, Holy Spirit, and I need You, Jesus and I need You, Abba. I need You all to be God with me, Immanuel. I do not want to go through this without all three of You, God, the Trinity. Please minister to my mind, will, emotions, body, soul, spirit and my heart. I pray for healing, even if You have to do some spiritual surgery to do it.

God spoke; not audibly but in a still small voice I hear with my heart.

"A lot of people out there are bipolar and they need to hear your story."

July Sunday PM 7-27-08

God spoke,

"What do you see?"

I told Him,"Pomegranates and bells as is in the temple."

God spoke,

"Your body is the temple of the Holy Spirit."

God spoke,

"What do you see?"

I told Him, "I see light and shadow. The shadow is turning to light."

God spoke to me,

"I can make the darkness into light. It may hurt. You may cry."

I told Him, "I am afraid of hurting."

God spoke to me,

"You have hurt all your life."

Abba, I thought of You, walking me through to the other side. When I go into depression, I have asked in the past that You walk me through it to the other side. It has always been a journey. You have not ever healed me right away. It has always been a process. It has never been the same way twice. But You, Abba have always brought me to the other side, back to a sound mind. Thank You and I praise You. In Jesus Name, Amen.

August Tuesday 8-19-08

This morning is the first time I praised God that I am manic-depressive called bipolar disorder. I thank Him for it. It led me into a relationship with Jesus, then Abba Father and then the Holy Spirit, God is three persons but one God. Sometimes it is still hard for me to grasp the concept. God is mystery. Does God answer all your questions? He does not answer all my questions, but it is enough for me that He knows all the answers. And He has the prerogative to not answer all my questions even when I meet Him in heaven. God is God. He answers me through a still, small, voice I cannot hear with my ears, but I think I hear Him with my heart. He also answers and speaks to me by His Holy Word the Bible and daily time reading God's Word in the Bible. He also answers through godly counsel. I prayed for godly counsel for years and years before God placed my pastor, Bro. Randy and his wife Pam in my life. Bro. Jim would come and visit me in the hospital and talk and pray with me, but he encouraged me to seek counsel with Bro. Randy.

Bro. Randy taught one Sunday night that Satan was my old landlord, but when Jesus saved me, God became my new LandLORD. But Satan intimidates me by keeping on showing up for me to serve him. Satan wants the "rent." But Bro. Randy says all we have to do when Satan shows up is tell him we are now under new management. You have to say it out loud because Satan cannot hear our thoughts.

Bro. Ted taught me how to not react to sin. Bro. Ted taught one Sunday years ago about what our response should be when we are tempted. He pretended to be dead. A dead person does not respond to anything going on around him. We do not have to sin, we have a choice to not respond.

Abba, Michael told me I do not even have to say the words out loud. Just pray to your big Brother Jesus for the LORD to rebuke Satan and his demons in a particular area you are having difficulty.

Abba, I do not have to speak the words out loud to have a critical tongue. They are my thoughts. It comes out more in my tone of voice. I do not have patience with some people. I do not have love for some people. I may not say the words I think out loud so others know what I think, but it comes out in my attitude. I have to live with my thoughts. I hear the arguing going on in my head. Things I would never say out loud play in my head. Some are Satan's and his demons' but a whole lot of it is years and years of just judging people by standards I cannot even live up to in the first place, so how can I expect someone else to? I do not want to sin against You anymore. And I do not have to. Satan may know how to push my buttons, but I do not have to respond! Not anymore, because Jesus lives in me and I am under new management! Forgive me and thank You for forgiving me. Thank You that You Father have prepared a place for the devil and his demons, they will be in hell forever. I praise You I thank You, I ask in Jesus Name, Amen.

From *Mission Mosaic*—Prayer Patterns

July Tuesday 7-1-08

And He looked up and saw the rich putting their gifts into the treasury, and He saw also a certain poor widow putting in two mites. So He said, "Truly I say to you that this poor widow has put in more than all; for all these out of their abundance have put in offerings for God, but she out of her poverty put in all the livelihood that she had." Luke 21:1-4 (NKJV)

And He (Jesus) saw also a certain poor widow putting in two mites.
Focus Verse: Luke 21:2 (NKJV)

Can you picture this scene with Jesus and His disciples taking place in your church? Where would they be sitting? Who would the different characters be? Are there ushers in the back of the sanctuary, counting up the envelopes? Any way the story is told. Jesus' remarks are shocking. Few churches would rather have an old woman dropping in two pennies than big celebrities dropping in thousands of dollars. Here, Jesus honors the witness of the poor woman, who was not ashamed to give the little bit that was all she had.

July Thursday 7-31-08

Abba, as best I know how, I give You all of me. In Jesus Name, Amen.

Again from that day's *Mission Mosaic*

Think about what you are giving to God. Is there one area in which you are sure you are giving all that you have? Perhaps that "all" looks like a tiny bit, compared to others' gifts, but read over the focus verse again. Jesus would much rather have a tiny bit, than an abundance of the leftovers.

July Thursday 7-31-08

I asked God, "Do I continue to work at the church cooking?" God spoke to me

"That is how you pay your tithe so you keep working."

I asked God "What would You have me give financially?"

God spoke to me

"Start giving now to the building fund. They may need more money to draw the plans. God is always right on time. People need to know they're worth it. You are worth it. You are worth the trouble."

(39)

Joy

August Friday 8-1-08
Daily Devotion from *Mission Mosaic*
James 1:2-4 Paraphrase mine: enter your name in the blanks.

> _____ *Count it all joy when you,*
> _____, *fall into various trials, knowing*
> *that the testing of* _____*'s faith produces*
> *patience. But let patience have its perfect work, that*
> *you,* _____, *may be perfect and complete,*
> *lacking nothing.* Based on James 1:2-4 (NKJV)

May Saturday (3:20 AM) 5-3-08

Definitions from *Webster's Encyclopedia Dictionary of the English Language*

Joy means:

great pleasure, gladness, delight, and rejoicing.

a thing which provokes delight: 'A thing of beauty is a joy for-ever.' (Keats, 'Endymion')

to take pleasure, rejoice in, to feel joy at: I joy to see you happy.

to give joy to, delight.

to enjoy

Count means:

a reckoning.

the number found by counting.

an item in an indictment, as, to be indicted on three counts.

to reckon by units in order to find a total.

to name the numerals in proper order.

to matter, play a part, as, your vote will count.

> *My brethren, count it all joy when you fall into various trials, knowing that the testing of your faith produces patience. But let patience have its perfect work, that you may be perfect and complete, lacking nothing. If any of you lacks wisdom, let him ask of God, who gives to all liberally and without reproach, and it will be given to him. But let him ask in faith, with no doubting, for he who doubts is like a wave of the sea driven and tossed by the wind. For let not that man suppose that he will receive anything from the Lord; he is a double-minded man, unstable in all his ways. James 1:2-8 (NKJV)*

*T*rials I am facing right now in my life:

Choosing between Jesus and a man.

Am I in love with going to church or am I in love with God?

Confusion.

Loss of memory.

I do not trust me and very few other people.

I have to cook next Saturday night Aug. 9 for the Steak and Shoot at church.

Teaching Sunday school to the three year olds.

Daddy has prostate cancer.

Jen, Jeff, Mackenzie and Lena

Jay, Melissa, Garrett, and Colby

Count it as "all joy" because of the result of trials, the testing of our faith. We are tested to be made strong, to be perfected. God is transforming us for eternity, not merely for this life. If this life were all I had, trials and hardships would serve no purpose and have no end but to embitter me.

Thank You LORD. That the result of trials is perfecting me, knowing You are transforming me is a reason for joy. In Jesus Name, Amen.

August Wednesday 8-20-08

Now I am what Dr. Wieck calls mixed mania. That is when you cycle from depression to manic back and forth and back and forth in a quick sequence of time. I am very much manic right now. It is hard to medicate since it changes so frequently. Sometimes I am manic, and I do things I should not. I become headstrong and do whatever I think of. Sometimes I destroy something I have made trying to make it "better." I have headstrong ideals even if they are wrong.

Abba, I am not worthy to be called Your daughter. I pray for a gentle Spirit. Forgive me that I am so headstrong. Pull me back into Your love and patience with me. Christ is the head over me. Help me trust You with all my decisions and reactions, especially when I am manic or depressed. Help me listen to godly counsel. Help me listen to You, God. Thank You Jesus and I pray for Your Holy Spirit's control over me. In Jesus Name, Amen.

(40)

There is Balance to Life

August Thursday 8-28-08 Meeting with Dr. Snowden 3:00 and again September Thursday 9-11-08 Meeting with Dr. Snowden 1:00

*A*bba, I see Dr. Snowden today. What do we talk about? Lots of things have happened. I again pray for a few simple words for him and myself; I pray for the best words and give us listening ears, his as well as mine. Help me listen to him and help me remember what has happened since we last met. Give us wisdom from You, LORD. I pray for godly wisdom, godly knowledge, godly understanding, godly revelation and godly discernment too. I pray to listen more than I talk today. Help me write down what he says so I will remember. Abba, I need nicknames for this book or else I need permission to use their real names. Help us in that process to know Your perfect will about the book, *Behind Closed Doors a journey through manic depression*. I need You more today than ever before. Teach me, I commit to You to learn.

Abba, Help me remember or help me forget. Bring to my remembrance the God moments of my life. Help me forget those things that are behind. I press on toward the mark of the high calling of Christ. In Jesus Name, Amen.

Not that I have already attained, or am already per-
fected; but I press on, that I may lay hold of that for
which Christ Jesus has also laid hold of me. Brethren,
I do not count myself to have apprehended; but one
thing I do, forgetting those things which are behind and
reaching forward to those things which are ahead, I
press toward the goal for the prize of the upward call of
God in Christ Jesus. Therefore let us, as many as are
mature, have this mind; and if in anything you think oth-
erwise, God will reveal even this to you. Nevertheless,
to the degree that we have already attained, let us
walk by the same rule, let us be of the same mind.
Philippians 3:12-16 (NKJV)

At my appointment with Dr. Snowden, he said there is balance to life:

Working   Resting
Loving   Playing

I have the "work" down pretty good, but I need to work on
love, rest and play. And I need to work on relationships.

We played = Daddy, Bro. Randy and I went fishing together,
then the next week Daddy and Momma, Bro. Randy, Pam and
I went fishing together. Pam caught ten fish. I caught two and
Daddy caught several. Momma cooked hamburgers and hot
dogs on the grill. Uncle Eddie and his work crew were building
a fence out at the pasture where we were; they came and ate
with us too. We had a good time and it was great being out
of the house and in the great outdoors. Thank You, Abba that
Daddy did not fall in either of the fires when he fell.

We played = usually we do not have time just to shop. We
are always buying groceries for the church and then straight
back home. It has been a very good day of just shopping.

Ministry = I am at the church now cooking what I can today
so it can be ready for tomorrow. Tomorrow I have to fix lunch for
two different places. Christian Woman's Job Corp is meeting

tomorrow, and I am suppose to furnish the green beans for them for lunch, and Bro. Jim has some special guests coming to hear him play the cowbells and sleigh bells and the saw. They are going to sing for us, and I am in charge of cooking for them. We are having stew, cornbread and dessert. Some of the people from our church are coming, too. And we are all going to eat lunch together. It will be fun.

I enjoy cooking. I like putting things together and seeing what comes out. And I like cooking for people. Without them I would not have a reason to cook. I put my headphones on and listen to praise and worship music and Jesus tells me what to do and when to do it and how to do it. I wish all days were like when I cook at the church. I just know God's leading on those days in a special way. It does not mean I do not sometimes burn things or the menu does not go as planned or that I do not sometimes get burned or cut. It is just I know His presence in the kitchen very definitely. I could not do what I do without Jesus. I would not be alive without Jesus. I want a relationship with Him like that all the time.

Tonight is not anything like I thought it would be. I am here in the church kitchen making cookies for Wednesday night fellowship. I am not alone here at the church. The Sky Hawks are meeting here tonight. That is a group of teenage boys who meet once a week for a devotional time. They come with food in hand but that is not why they meet. They meet because they had revival this summer when they went to camp, and they do not want to lose it. They meet to fellowship, but also for one of them to lead the Bible study and a time of prayer.

I have been crucified with Christ; it is no longer I who live, but Christ lives in me; and the life which I now live in the flesh I live by faith in the Son of God, who loved me and gave Himself for me. Galatians 2:20 (NKJV)

Abba, I know how they feel. I do not want to lose this either. I want relationship with You, God. I do not want to be alone again without You in my life—not for a day, or an hour or a minute, or even a second. I need You desperately, all the time. How do I put it into words what You did and continue to do for me? I was as good as dead, before You came to live in me. I could not feel anything, but pain, sorrow, hurt and abandonment. I was so full of sin before You saved me, forgave me and started the process of cleansing me. I had a hard heart. Do not ever stop changing me — even if it hurts, do not stop working on me. Now I live, yet, not I but You, the very Son of God, live through me. I do not ever want it any other way. I ask all to Your glory and praise LORD Jesus, Amen.

September 11:04 PM Friday 9-12-08

Abba, thank You, I did not plan one thing today. This day was all Your doing and I had a blast. I had my quiet time with You this morning. I organized all my scrapbooking stuff, so I can start working on a faithbook for Garrett, then Colby and then Lena. I also need to do a vacation scrapbook. I also need to do a personal testimony faithbook. I have already done a faithbook for Mackenzie. Help me; I do not want to do it alone. I need Your help God. I ask in the Holy Name of Jesus, Amen.

It was not hard to organize the faithbooking materials. I just separated everything into a bag marked with what was in it: Trash, Sunday school, Boston, Saint Louis, family reunion, Australia, Okinawa, and VBS. I organized my faithbooking bags and marked them with post a notes and masking tape. I even had time to lie down and rest a few minutes before it was time to go to the party and the football game. My band director, Mr. Raeke, was celebrating 50 years as a teacher, band director and community servant. I had the privilege of thanking him for letting me play in the band. I never learned how to play my clarinet while I was in band. The only thing I knew how to play was "Rebel Rouser" which he wrote. He still let me stay in the band. Anyway, the alumni were invited to attend a party with Mr. Raeke. After we visited in the building, we then went over to the football field to participate with the cheerleaders. It was mostly past cheerleaders, mascots, drum majors, twirlers and flags. But because I was in band, I wanted to go, too. Momma was a twirler when she was in high school, so I went with her.

Abba, You showed me how much You love me tonight. You reserve the right to answer prayers long after we have given up even asking. Tonight You answered my teenage prayer; You let me be on the field during the entire football game, cheering on our Bearcats. We hardly ever go to a game, so it was very special. I tried out to be cheerleader as a teenager and as long as I was with the group I was okay, but when I tried out solo—I froze and then ran off the gym floor. Some of my friends voted for me anyway, but I did not make the squad. Thank You, I was not afraid tonight. It was pure joy. I took all the pictures I wanted. Momma, Jen and I bought alumni T-shirts. Momma and I even received cheerleading medals. You showed me tonight it is okay to play. I thank You and I praise You—You orchestrated the whole day and night and I had a blast. I ask in the most Precious Name I know, Jesus, Amen.

I want to play by doing faithbooking, which was created by Denise Jordon. She introduced me to the book, *God Moments* by Alan D. Wright. Alan D. Wright encourages us to write down what God has done in our lives:

Amazing Rescue: begin with childhood memories or recall the moment of near-accidents or life-threatening circumstances you survived. Pay particular attention to illnesses from which you have recovered. All healing is a rescue. Spiritual benefit: peace

Holy Attraction: a moment when God led you toward a healthier path, enabled you to resist a temptation, or inspired you to take the high road. Remember where you were when you did not obey or opt for purity, remember times when you opted out for purity-not giving in to temptation, choosing good friends, giving money to charity, helping others. Spiritual benefit: renewed obedience

Unearned Blessings: a moment when God gave you an unexpected blessing or an undeserved gift. When your skills were inadequate but you were blessed anyway — treasures in your life such as people you love and who love you, places that have molded you, provisions that came in timely or unexpected ways; promotions you have been given; privileges you have enjoyed. Spiritual benefit: lasting joy

Revealed Truth: is a moment when God spoke to you through the Bible, inner peace, wise counsel, or a God-inspired message. When has a verse or theme of scripture come alive to you? When have you said, "A light bulb just went on in my mind? When have you just known what you were supposed to do? Spiritual benefit: renewed confidence

Valuable Adversity: a moment in which God sustained you in a difficult time or made you stronger through the test of adversity or an adversity that saved you from worse destruction or prepared you to receive a greater blessing. Our most difficult moments may be some of our greatest God moments. Spiritual benefit: perseverance

Do not forget the things your eyes have seen or let them slip from your heart. Exodus 13:9-10 (NKJV)

Remember… Deuteronomy 5:15 (NKJV)

Remember how the LORD led you. Deuteronomy 8:2 (NKJV)

Remember the LORD your God, for it is He who gives you the ability to produce wealth. Deuteronomy 8:18 (NKJV)

I will remember your miracles of long ago. I will meditate on all your works. Psalm 77:11-12 (NKJV)

Praise the LORD, O my soul, and forget not all His benefits—who forgives all your sins and heals all your diseases, who redeems your life from the pit... Psalm 103:2 (NKJV)

He has made His wonderful works to be remembered; Psalm 111:4 (NKJV)

Do not be afraid of them. Remember the LORD. Nehemiah 4:14 (NKJV)

Remember the LORD in a distant land. Jeremiah 51-50 (NKJV)

Don't you remember the five loaves for the 5,000? Matthew 16:9 (NKJV)

I will always remind you of these things...I think it is right to refresh your memory. 2 Peter 1:12 (NKJV)

Experiencing God: God is always at work around you!
Things only God can do:

God draws people to Himself. (when you see someone come to Christ)
God causes people to seek after Him. (when people are asking about spiritual matters)
God reveals spiritual truth. (when you understand the Bible or a verse)
God convicts the world of guilt regarding sin. (when you experience conviction in regards to sin)

God convicts the world of righteousness. (when you are being convicted of the righteousness of Christ)
God convicts the world of judgment. (when you are being convicted of judgment)

Faithbooking benefits

Glorifies God
Builds your faith
Leaves a Spiritual legacy

When I would clean my room at home, Momma would tell me to "Keep it clean." Innocently enough spoken then, but every time I ever cleaned my house after that, even to this day, I hear Satan echo those words in my head, "Keep it clean" and I cannot. I do not know how, but I am learning. I simply pick up and clean up as I go along. I do not tackle a whole house or even a whole room. I start with a corner that needs it the most and day by day keep at it.

Jen taught me about the bags. One says keep, one says throw away, and one says give away. There can be more bags than that. I keep one bag marked Sunday school. I teach the three year olds at our church. I always have to take something to Sunday school. I keep a bag for the church kitchen because I wash and take back to the church the clean dish towels, dish rags and aprons. Keeping the bags separated helps. So name your bags and write on them with a sharpie. It keeps me from having to go back through the bags if I mark them, so I do not get confused.

I have asked God to help me. Instead of stacking clean laundry on the bed, it goes into the drawers or hung up in the closet. Instead of piling laundry up in my room and never knowing what was clean or dirty, I have a place where it goes until I do laundry. I need to invest in a laundry sorter of some kind so they could be separated as I put them in that place, but that will come. Instead of piling clean clothes that I could wear again on the totes at the end of my bed, I hang them back up. Do you see what I mean about cleaning as you go instead of having to have a marathon of cleaning to do before company comes? And now I throw things away. So if I have a piece of trash, it goes in the trash bag right away, so I do not have to go through it again later.

Momma said I could mess up every dish in the kitchen when I cooked and I did. I did not like to wash dishes with hard caked on food I had to scrub off. The solution to that is rinsing as I finish cooking and eating that meal. Rinse it off right then before it gets hard or if something is already hard, put some dishwashing soap in it and hot water and let it soak until the next meal and rinse it then. Load the dishwasher after each meal or as soon as something gets put in the sink.

Even my mail stacked up on the kitchen table. The Crown Financial Ministries Seminar taught me to pay bills as they come in. Deal with it then and there and do not put it off. That way you only have to deal with it one time and trash either goes in the trash or the shredder so it does not pile up.

That is some of what God is teaching me about cleaning. God has taught me also not to go very long before asking Him if there is any sin in my life. Quickly come to Him and ask for forgiveness. I want to be the fastest repenter on earth and turn away from that sin and not to do it anymore. When we ask for forgiveness from God and turn away from sin, that is called repentance and God puts our sin as far as the east is from the west. If you go north, you go to the North Pole, and then you go south until you run into the South Pole. You can go east around the globe forever or you can go west forever. How far is your sin from you?

> *As far as the east is from the west, So far has He removed our transgressions from us.* Psalm 103:12 (NKJV)

Abba, in the past when I reorganized and cleaned my room, I would move things to a new spot and then I would go back to find it in the original spot, only it was not there anymore. It got so bad I was afraid to move anything from where it was. But God—I have learned You know where I put things. All I have to do is ask You where it is. And then all I have to do is be obedient to Your leading. You do not always lead me right to it. You see if I am going to be obedient to Your still small voice in the first place and then You show me what I lost. Thank You for answered prayers. I am smiling again. I praise You God for healing me. Thank You I am not afraid anymore. In Jesus' blessed Name above all names, Amen.

(41)

Praying For Such a Little Thing

October (Sunday, written after church) 10-3-04

*I*t may seem like such a little thing to you, but I needed a praying mantis for my Sunday school class today. In class and worship today we studied the *40 Days of Purpose* by Rick Warren. But we have to go back two weeks. Last week we were studying bugs, how God made us for a purpose—the way we are for a reason. I thought a praying mantis insect would be great to show the children. I did not know that this week we would focus in on just the praying mantis. So I prayed and searched one night between midnight and 3:00 am. I found lots of great bugs that were just what I needed for the class. I looked last Saturday during the day and caught more great bugs and even a baby frog. But I kept reminding God that I thought a praying mantis would be so much better. But I did not find one. The class was a great success that Sunday. The children loved all the bugs. And we learned: God made us what and who we are. By the way, I love collecting bugs. I had so much fun with these lessons. And we shared our bugs with the two year old class too.

Then came time to start preparing for this Sunday, the lesson did not come together as it did the week before. I even called Bobbie and she helped me a lot. She always is such a support to me. This week's lesson features a praying mantis, so I kept praying and asking God because I really did need the little insect this week. I did not search all week for one. I knew if I caught him early he might die and I did not want a dead one — I wanted a live one. Saturday came and I woke up late. I had to go to Margaret's house to pick up all of the flower arrangements from the garage sale for the church. She said Momma could have all the material. That was another answer to prayer. I do not remember what else I did, but I did not have time to look for a bug. That afternoon the LORD impressed me to go looking. I went, at first, without a jar to catch him — O ye of little faith. But I went back in the house and grabbed the plastic jar I had used last week to hold the bugs. I walked out the door, praying, "God I really need a praying mantis this week for Sunday school and I do not have all day to spend looking for him like I did last week."

A cool front had come through that brought an inch and a half of rain which was another answer to prayer. You see we have only had to water one time during this whole summer. Sometimes our water bill is $300.00 a month, but not this summer. I praise and thank God. But back to the bug, I walked out the door, turned to my right, walked down the sidewalk and was noticing that the hydrangea had some more flowers on it. I looked at three on my right and then to the one right in front of me. There was a big, gray praying mantis. We did not even need the magnifying glass like we did last week to be able to see the bugs I caught. He was the most beautiful thing I had ever seen. He was beautiful because God heard my prayer and answered so specifically. God had not provided him the week before when I really did not need him. God's answer then was "wait." God answered in His perfect timing, and I did not even have any trouble catching him.

Abba, I praise You, LORD, Thank You God for listening and answering me and so the children could see up close and personal one of Your creations that "worships" You. I ask in Jesus precious name, Amen.

November (written Sunday after church) 11-8-09

I looked in my faithbooking supplies and found the above journaling I had done about five years ago. As I read it, I realized I again needed a praying mantis to take to the three year olds at Sunday school because we were studying prayer again all month long and they are just learning to pray without our help. I prayed again to catch another praying mantis. Another cool front had come through. I looked on the hydrangea bush but there were no flowers or bugs. I looked on the honeysuckle vines, the tomato bushes, the pepper plants, the squash and okra plants and found nothing but grasshoppers. I found strawberries on the plants in the garden and ate all I could reach. Then I searched the apricot trees in the orchard and found nothing. Then I headed back to the hydrangea bushes and looked over by the crepe myrtles. There on the white brick around the window of the house was a praying mantis. I put the jar over it and he crawled in. It is marvelous to see the variety God made even in His insects. God created each of us and we are all different and unique. Even twins have their own set of fingerprints, special only to each person. God answers prayer, even little prayers that do not mean anything to anyone else. God wants a relationship with us; not just saved but an ongoing daily walk every day that we live. Each new day is different, unique and special because God is never boring. God shows up big when we ask Him.

When Jesus died on the cross to pay our sin penalty, He died for us. Trust Him today. He cares for you. God loved you so much He gave His only begotten Son to save you. Jesus rose again and lived on earth for forty days before He went back to heaven. Then He sent the Holy Spirit to indwell us so we would never again have to be alone. Jesus can be with every believer through His Holy Spirit. Ask to be filled with His Holy Spirit. The Holy Spirit makes all the difference in living for Jesus in our world today.

Abba, I praise You, LORD. The children had fun looking at the praying mantis at Sunday school. It is amazing to watch the children mature, grow and learn about You, Jesus, the Holy Spirit and Your Word during Sunday school in the years that we have them in class. Thank You that You listen to even our smallest prayer concerns. Thank You that You answer prayer in Your perfect timing. Thank You that You always listen to us. I did not tell anyone else what I needed as I looked for the praying mantis. It was cool that day and most insects were in hiding but God, You again provided what I needed. I thank You for meeting my needs for that is one way You show that You love us. In Jesus Blessed Name, Amen.

(42)

What Helps

A heating pad on my back or neck because my muscles are so tense and I cannot relax.
Stretching exercises
Hot chamomile caffeine free herbal tea at bedtime with a little sugar in it.
A real hot bath anytime of the day and just soak and relax and not have to rush.
Whether I am manic or depressed walking helps, any kind of exercise would help to use up some of this manic energy. Walking helps the brain chemicals work the right way whether manic or depressed.
Praying always helps, not only praying for myself but also praying for others. Just talking to God helps; it does not have to be big important things but also the littlest things. He is always listening. He is always active and answering behind the scenes and sometimes He lets me in on what He is doing. Enlist others to pray for you too and keep asking until you are better.
Knowing my Abba Father and Jesus and the Holy Spirit are praying for me right now is always a great comfort to me.
Talking about it helps.
Getting still and listening to God helps and then obey what He says.

Reading the Bible helps unless I am full blown manic and then I do not read the Bible because then it does not make sense and I read all sorts of things into it that should not be there. I take it out of context, so there have been times in my life when I have had to put the Bible down for a time or season until the manic subsides. I have scriptures written on cards in my bathroom and in my purse and it helps me to stop and read them.

Writing this down helps. It is helping me, and I pray for those reading this, that it helps you too.

It helps to know Abba as my Father, my DADDY.

It helps to know Jesus as my big Brother, my King, my LORD, my Savior, my Husband to be and my Best Friend in the whole world.

It helps getting to know the Holy Spirit as my Comforter, my Counselor and my Helper.

Going to church helps. Find a Bible believing and preaching and praying church. Keep looking until you find a church that loves you and where you can love them in return.

It is helpful to have encouraging people around me.

Hugs help and I have learned the best way you can get a hug is to give someone a hug and sometimes they hug back.

Quiet helps because in the quiet I hear God.

Listening to Christian music helps me praise God while I am going through the trials of this life. God has a purpose and a plan for good and not for evil to give a future and a hope based on Jeremiah 29:11. Is our God a good God? Trust Him. Is He helping? Believe Him. Obey God's leading. And praise and thank God now.

For I know the thoughts that I think toward you, says the LORD, thoughts of peace and not of evil, to give you a future and a hope. Then you will call upon Me and go and pray to Me, and I will listen to you. And you will seek Me and find Me, when you search for Me with all your heart. I will be found by

you, says the LORD, and I will bring you back from your captivity; I will gather you from all the nations and from all the places where I have driven you, says the LORD, and I will bring you to the place from which I cause you to be carried away captive.
Jeremiah 29:11-14 (NKJV)

*E*xamples of what I have been listening to on my head-phones are: Ayiesha Woods, Chris Tomlin, Natalie Grant, Niclole C. Mullen, Tommy Walker, Women of Faith, Curt Coffield, Casting Crowns, Stephen Curtis Chapman, Dallas Holmes and Twila Paris.

It helps to have the right music going on in my head all the time. That happens as I sing praise and worship music to God. As I memorize the songs by singing them over and over again, God then can bring a song to my mind; I really listen to the words and sing it with all my heart back to Him.

Just to sit or stand still helps. I move from one foot to the other, it is a side effect of one of my medicines. I call it "stutter steppin". But I have noticed I do not do it during the church service.

Be still, and know that I am God; I will be exalted among the nations, I will be exalted in the earth!
Psalm 46:10 (NKJV)

It helps to get on my knees or on my face before God, if you cannot God understands.
Knowing that God is God and not me helps.
Memorizing scripture helps.
Learning about bipolar disorder helps.
If you can find a Christian psychiatrist and Christian psychologist helps.
It helps to have a Christian Counselor.
Family helps.
It helps to take a multi vitamin every morning. I noticed this when I was pregnant both times with my children. I

never felt better than when I was pregnant with both of them and taking my pre-natal vitamins. I do not know how long I have taken vitamins, maybe the last five years, but they help.

It helps to take calcium.

It helps to take Omega 3 fish oil soft gels. If you take the ones that are enteric coated you do not burp the fish taste all day. I get mine at Sam's. I take 1000 mg in the morning and 1000 mg at night, it helps my memory which is a big issue with me and it helps my mood.

It helps to have a gallon Ziploc bag to put all your medicines in so you can take them with you when you see your doctors, psychiatrist and psychologist. They all need to know everything you are taking all the way down to an aspirin.

It helps to have a pill dispenser with morning, noon, evening, and night separated and a whole week's worth of pills loaded into one contained pill box, you can buy one at the pharmacy department of the drug store.

Silence helps but a fan going in the room with you helps drown out the noises that go bump in the night.

It helps to be around people who encourage me and lift me up out of just being by myself and with my own thoughts if the thoughts aren't so good.

It helps to have other caring people listening to you, people who love you despite the storm of depression or manic; people who know what you are like and will pray hard until you are back to that point.

It helps to be anointed with oil and for people to lay hands on you and pray just for you and your situation even if that situation is a sin you just cannot get victory, without God's help.

It helps to pray with people—you pray and let them pray too. It helps to pray for other people who need your prayer support.

It helps to read an entire book, like the book of John, in the Bible at a time and then read it again. Then it helps to read it one verse of scripture at a time so you do not get confused. Ask God hard tough questions and easy ones too. God will answer your questions if you will wait on Him and tell Him you are listening. It helps to write down in a journal what God tells you so you do not forget.

Fasting helps. But I had to learn some lessons the hard way. God understands we have to take our medicines. So do not skip taking them. If you have to take them with food, eat some saltine crackers to take them, God still honors the fast. Fasting can be many things:

Fast from watching TV
Fast from listening to radio or music
Fast from cursing
Fast from drinking any fluids except water
Fast from talking
Fast from food

I have to make a warning here: You do not stop drinking water completely. You have to have water to survive. And Jesus loves you too much and can help you learn to really live again. He needs you to stay alive and serve Him. Hold on to Him. Grab hold of God. Cling to Him. He will hold you.

It helps to quit drinking alcohol and beer. Jesus can help you stop.

It helps to not ever start abusing drugs. Jesus can help you stop if you are.

It helps to drink decaffeinated teas and coffees while you are manic.

It helps to drink caffeinated drinks when you are depressed but only in the mornings, if you drink them too late in the day you will not be able to sleep at night...

It helps just to talk to God, maybe not even about problems, but just tell Him how your day is going. Praise Him and thank Him. We are to give thanks in all things. We are to pray about everything. Tell Him you love Him.

giving thanks always for all things to God the Father in the name of our Lord Jesus Christ, Ephesians 5:20A (NKJV)

Abba, teach us to fast. Help us seek Your will about when to fast and how long to fast and when to stop fasting. Help us read Your Word the Bible, the Bread of Life, when we fast. Help us come to Your Word a little bit hungry. Let Your Word feed us. Help us be sensitive as we pray to You. Give us the right words to pray. LORD, teach us to pray. Talking to God, listening to God and then obeying what You have told us to do. Give us Your faith to believe in Jesus and You, Abba Father and the Holy Spirit. In Jesus Name, Amen.

August Friday AM 8-1-08
From the Daily Devotional—*Daily Moments in His Presence* by Frances J. Roberts
Endurance—from On the Highway of surrender

Now hope does not disappoint, because the love of God has been poured out in our hearts by the Holy Spirit who was given to us. Romans 5:5 (NKJV)

These words are on the page—God spoke them over me

"My child, do not flinch under My disciplines. I never send more than you can endure. Can you accept the cup of suffering as readily as you embrace joy? You can do so in greater degrees as your trust in Me increases. My love never fails, even when it brings you pain. It is in the patient endurance of affliction that the soul is seasoned with grace. It is a barren life that holds only happiness. Saints are not nurtured by levity. Hope does not spring from good fortune.

...For He Himself has said, "I will never leave you nor forsake you." Hebrews 13:5 (NKJV)

Abba, I reread Pat's notes of the Beth Moore seminar last night: faith, hope, love and the greatest of these is love. If I do not do anything else in life, I pray to love You, Abba Father, Jesus and Holy Spirit, but I pray others will know how much I love You by how much I love them. I pray for love. Your love never fails. Help me not to flinch or get sad or depressed under Your disciplines or trials. You will not send more than I can endure, and You will provide a way of escape from temptation. I pray for huge patience and huge faith in You. I pray for the hope only you can give. Thank You for Your grace. I pray for joy in the journey with You. I need You Holy Spirit. I surrender to You. I need You Abba, my DADDY, and I need You Jesus. I surrender to You. I submit to You, I pray You will sanctify me. I pray for self-control by Your Holy Spirit's control. But I could still use work on this sin. I am short with people when I feel irritable. Sometimes I just ignore people that bother me. Forgive me for judging people. I do not want to judge others anymore. I am sorry. People are so important to You; help them be important to me, too. Help me find a balance between doing what others expect of me and what You would have me do. Help me not to be irritable with people. When they need an answer right away, I pray for Your wisdom, knowledge, understanding, revelation, sound judgment and discernment. Help me with people; I do not do well in relationships. I pray fill me, Holy Spirit, with Your love and compassion for all people.

Abba, why do I just know You are with me sometimes more than other times? You never leave me nor forsake me. Am I the one who leaves You? Or is there just something different about being in Your house, the church? I would rather be in church than anywhere else on earth. And that is good because I am there a lot. I love what You do through me. I love Your touch. I may not be able to feel it with my body, but I sense it in my heart, soul and spirit. You are so different from what I thought You were like at first as a child. I thought You were an ogre and mean. But You are not like that at all. You are love. You, God, may be big, but You are personal. You meet my needs. You complete me. I praise You for all three of You—

Abba my DADDY; Jesus my LORD and King and Husband to be; and God the Holy Spirit. There really would not be room enough to write all the ways You love me. All the books in the world cannot contain You. When I ask You to show me Your love, You "blow my mind." I was so afraid of asking You to do that. It is a prayer of Beth Moore I learned in Bible study one time. I am not afraid of it anymore. Please "blow my mind" with Your Word.

You do not ever overpower me when You empower me by Your Holy Spirit. You make me more than I can be on my own. Do not ever quit. Do not ever stop even if it hurts. Sorrows come even for Christians. But, it is better now going through it with You. I do not know how to explain the difference in my life since I came into a relationship with You. I do not want to live without You. Thank You that I do not have to live without You Jesus. In Jesus Name, Amen.

This helped—Margaret August (Friday) 8-22-08

If God brings you to it,

He will bring you through it

Happy moments, praise God

Difficult moments, seek God

And praise Him and thank Him anyway

Quiet moments (turn off the cell phone,

get someone else to answer the phone,

or just let the answering machine pick it up)

Make some quiet moments to worship God

Painful moments trust God

Every moment thank God

Jesus can help you.

Tell Him your problem

He already knows all about it.

But He wants to hear it from your viewpoint

He wants to hear your heart.

(43)

This Information Helped

Diagnosis

*I*f you think you may have bipolar disorder, you are not alone. Bipolar disorder is estimated to affect millions of American adults each year. Yet for many people with the disease, accurate diagnosis, and therefore, appropriate treatment, may be delayed for years.

Bipolar disorder is a condition that can cause extreme swings in mood—from manic highs to depressive lows. To be diagnosed with bipolar disorder you must have experienced a high period (mania or hypomania). However, most people with bipolar disorder when ill or when symptomatic experience more lows than highs. These lows are known as bipolar depression—and they can consume you. Your health care professional is trained to make a correct diagnosis based on your symptoms and a careful review of your medical history.

Bipolar mania is an "extreme high" mood. During a manic high, people feel unusually great. It is common to be overly talkative, have lots of energy, and need little sleep.

Hypomania is a less severe form of mania—but it is no less important to report to your health care professional. One of the ways you can be sure to get an accurate diagnosis is to talk to your health care professional about all the symptoms you are experiencing or have experienced in the past, including any manic or hypomanic episodes.

Impact of Bipolar Disorder

- Bipolar disorder may make it harder to get along with others and have good relationships
  - o Divorce rates, for example, are almost 2 to 3 times higher for people with bipolar disorder than for people without it
  - o Holding down a job, completing an education, taking care of children, and managing money may also be more difficult
- Bipolar disorder may make drinking too much alcohol or abusing drugs more likely
  - o It may cause you to take risks that could cause harm to yourself
- The depressive symptoms, also called bipolar depression, can be extremely disruptive to a person's life

Misdiagnosis is common

Many patients with bipolar disorder initially seek treatment for depressive symptoms. Unfortunately, the diagnosis of bipolar disorder is oftentimes missed. One of the ways to help get an accurate diagnosis is to talk to your health care professional about all the symptoms you are experiencing, including any manic symptoms or hypomanic symptoms (hypomania is a less severe form of mania).

The symptoms of major depressive disorder, also called depression, are similar to the symptoms of bipolar depression. In a national survey, more than two-thirds of people with bipolar disorder were originally misdiagnosed with other disorders. And over one-third of people with bipolar disorder who were originally misdiagnosed waited 10 years or more before receiving an accurate diagnosis.

If you have unresolved depressive symptoms caused by bipolar disorder—or if you think it is possible you've been misdiagnosed with major depressive disorder—be sure to talk to your health care professional about all the symptoms you are experiencing, including any manic or hypomanic episodes. Here are some tips for working with your health care professional to assist him or her in making your diagnosis.

- Keep accurate records and notes so that you can have a productive conversation with your health care professional
  o Consider using a Mood Tracking Diary to keep track of your symptoms
- Tell your health care professional if you have a history of mania or hypomania
- Tell your health care professional if you have a family history of bipolar disorder

Bipolar Depression Symptoms

For some patients with bipolar disorder, the depressive symptoms, also called bipolar depression, can be more disabling than the manic symptoms. It is important that you discuss all your symptoms with your health care professional, including any manic episodes. The depressive symptoms of bipolar disorder are similar to, and in fact often misdiagnosed as, symptoms of major depressive disorder, also called depression. To be diagnosed with bipolar disorder you must have experienced a high period of either mania or hypomania (a less severe form of mania). So be sure to talk to your health care professional about all the symptoms you are experiencing, including any manic episodes. This will assist your health care professional in recognizing the differences between these often-similar disorders.

Symptoms of Bipolar Depression

Sadness

- Feelings of worthlessness
- Losing interest in things and activities you once enjoyed
- Being overcome by feelings of guilt, failure, and hopelessness
- Becoming sad and unable to concentrate, remember things, or even make simple decisions
- Experiencing physiological changes like differences in appetite or weight, energy levels, and sleep schedules
- Possibly thinking about death or suicide, in extreme cases

What is bipolar mania?

A manic or hypo manic episode is what separates a diagnosis of major depressive disorder, also called depression, from bipolar disorder. Bipolar mania is an "extreme high" mood. During a manic high, people feel unusually great. It is common to be overly talkative, have lots of energy, and need little sleep. Hypomania is a less severe form of mania, but it is no less important to report to your doctor.

Talk to your doctor if you think you have had, or may be having, a manic episode. Discuss all the symptoms you may be feeling.

Symptoms of Bipolar Mania Include

- Feeling unusually great and launching into several new projects at once
- Sleeping a lot less, acting more fidgety, and talking much more
- Mixing up thoughts and being easily distracted
- Taking unnecessary risks
- Going to extremes sexually, financially, and socially

- Bipolar mania can be disruptive. However, like bipolar depression, bipolar mania can be treated effectively.

Some of the Goals of Bipolar Disorder Treatment

- Reduce symptoms of depressive episodes
- Reduce symptoms of manic episodes
- Reduce the likelihood of future episodes/relapse
- Reduce the severity of the disease
- Provide assistance and support to patients and family

If a Loved One Has a Mental Illness...

Strong relationships are important and can have a significant impact on people with depression or bipolar disorder. Be patient when communicating with your loved one. Here are additional things to consider.

- Stay connected. Work with your loved one and his or her health care professional
- Try to be understanding. Let your loved one approach life at his or her own pace, and avoid expecting too much or too little
- Remind yourself that your loved one is suffering from a chronic mental illness that is causing your loved one to act as he or she does. Do not blame him or her, just like you would not if a physical disorder were causing your loved one to change

Supporting your loved one

If you have a family member or friend with major depressive disorder, also called depression, or with bipolar disorder, it is important to watch for and try to prevent suicidal thoughts and actions. Make sure to:

- pay close attention to any changes, especially sudden changes, in mood, behaviors, thoughts, or feelings. This is very important when an antidepressant medicine is started or when the dose is changed
- call the health care provider right away to report new or sudden changes in mood, behavior, thoughts, or feelings
- keep all follow-up visits with the health care provider as scheduled. Call the health care provider between visits as needed, especially if there are concerns about symptoms
- Here are some additional things you should know and ways you can help.

Understanding bipolar disorder

People with bipolar disorder will have times when their mood is "normal" and balanced, or close to that. But they will also have times of extreme mood swings. These are called "episodes."

Although it may sound strange, your loved one could be experiencing an episode and not even realize it. You should familiarize yourself with the warning signs of a depressed "low" or manic "high," and you can aid your loved one by letting his or her health care professional know right away when you detect a warning sign.

Whether you are the spouse, a significant other, a family member, or a close friend of someone with bipolar disorder, your support is important. There are a few basic things you may be able to do to assist your loved one in managing bipolar disorder. Understanding the condition and its signs and symptoms is an important one.

Help with medical appointments

It is important for your loved one to keep scheduled medical appointments. This is true during episodes of illness and even when your loved one is not having symptoms. If you are a spouse or significant other, you should consider attending medical appointments with your loved one's permission to receive information firsthand from the health care professional.

Remind your loved one about medical appointments and offer to give him or her support during the appointment or to provide transportation, as needed.

Help with medication

Your loved one may not want to take prescribed medication. Side effects may be a concern. Do what you can, within reason, to enable your loved one to discuss the need for medication with his or her health care professional promptly. The health care professional should promptly be told about the following concerns.

- If your loved one is complaining about side effects
- If your loved one does not think a medication is working the way it should
- If your loved one stops or is thinking about stopping taking a prescribed medication

Plan for future bipolar disorder episodes

Having a plan in place may let you and your loved one feel a little more in control. Make arrangements with your loved one during stable periods to help reduce problems during future episodes of illness. Talk about the possible need to put certain safeguards in place. These safeguards might include taking away credit cards, banking privileges, and car keys, and having a plan about when to go to the hospital.

Make sure you know where to find the following things.

- Contact information for your loved one's health care professionals and pharmacy

- A list of your loved one's medications and dosages
- Your loved one's insurance information, such as plan names, coverage, and approved providers
- Contact information for bipolar disorder support groups or crisis lines
- I found this information off of the website:

www.seroquelxr.com/bipolar-disorder

There are charts and forms that can be copied and used to keep track of all the things you need to write down for your records, they are found at the above website.

(44)

One Step Upon Another

For we do not have a High Priest who cannot sympathize with our weaknesses, but was in all points tempted as we are, yet without sin. Hebrews 4:15 (NKJV)

Jesus died on the cross to pay our sin penalty with His life and His own blood. Jesus, You loved us to death. Thank You is not enough, but it is what You ask of us, so I thank You and praise You for saving me. I praise You Jesus that You came back to life. Thank You that our last breath on earth is our first breath in heaven.

It is so simple a little child can do it. We have to come to God in childlike faith believing He will do the work in us that needs to be done.

Some people are afraid of becoming a Christian. Not knowing what to expect is their greatest fear. I just wanted to calm some of those fears. It is the most important decision you will ever make. You need Him more than you will ever know. Do not wait for something bad to happen to need God.

The first step after asking God to save us is telling someone else, maybe someone you know who prays for you. Tell them that Jesus saved you and tell them how. How God saved you is your testimony. You are the only one in the world with your testimony. It is yours, but it belongs to God too. You see He orchestrated the whole thing and He gives you the faith to believe. So each time you tell someone what Christ Jesus did in your life it gives the glory to God. That is where the glory always belongs.

Another step of faith is finding a Bible teaching and preaching church to attend where you can learn more about this God you too can now call Abba Father because He has now become your DADDY. Beth Moore says Abba means DADDY; He can be your DADDY too.

"I will be a Father to you, And you shall be My sons and daughters, says the LORD Almighty." 2 Corinthians 6:18 (NKJV)

You join a church by walking down to the front of the church and take the pastor's hand and tell him that either you are already saved by trusting in Jesus to save you or else if you have not done that yet, he can lead you in that process and that step of obedience to Christ Jesus.

Another step of faith is believer's baptism by immersion. Immersion means a pastor is going to dip your body in water. You can hold your nose; it is all right everybody does. The pastor brings you right back up immediately. He says something like the words Bro. Randy says, "I baptize you my brother or sister (as the case may be) in Christ, in the Name of the Father, the Son and the Holy Spirit. Buried with Him in baptism, we are raised to walk in newness of life." Baptism pictures the death, burial, and resurrection of Christ Jesus our LORD. Baptism is not essential to be saved, but it is your step of obedience that tells the others in church that you are a believer in Christ and that is called your public profession of faith in Christ Jesus.

August Monday 8-18-08

Another step of faith is to get a Bible. I like the New King James Version because it has all the Names of God capitalized including when God is referred to as He, His, My, or Me; it just helps make things clearer and easier to understand. It also has all the verses in it unlike so many of the other Bible translations out on the market. Always ask God to bless the reading of His Word just like a blessing said before a meal. Just as an example:

Abba, I ask Your blessing upon the reading of Your Word. Speak to my heart as only You can as only You want to and as only You will to. Spirit of truth lead me to all truth. Thank You, Your Word is truth. In Jesus Name, Amen.

Simply ask God to speak to You through His Word the Bible. The Billy Graham Training Center Bible in New King James Version is very easy to understand and has great notes in it to help you understand the scriptures. The Bible is divided up into 66 books. It is all written in red. The Old Testament looks forward to Calvary and the New Testament looks back at Calvary. Calvary is when Jesus died on the cross to pay our sin penalty. The Bible is God's love letter to us, so read it daily. The 66 books of the Bible are divided up into books, chapters and also individual verses, but in the original scrolls there were no chapters or verses separating the Bible. In fact there are some places in Ephesians where there were not even any periods separating many, many, many verses. They were all one sentence. Do not worry about not knowing how to look up the scriptures and finding the books of the Bible. That will come with time as you spend time at home reading what God has to say to you, so invest in a good Bible. Bibles with the tabs of the names of the books of the Bible help to find what you want to look up or look on the index page in the front of your Bible that tells where the page number of the different books that are in your Bible.

Another step of obedience is to pray. Ask God to teach you to pray. It is like breathing in and out. You talk to God and ask Him to talk to you. Tell God you are listening and ask Him to help you recognize His voice. It is a still small voice so get very quiet and still and allow God to speak to you. When He answers, obey what He tells you to do. Part of prayer is thanking Him and praising God. A whole lot of it is just getting quiet and still enough to hear His voice. He never yells or tells you to do something contrary to the scriptures. If you hear something like that, it is not God at all. God is very patient. It takes time. It is a journey with Him, walking with Him through this life day by day and into eternity in heaven with Him. Some day Jesus is coming back to get His Bride the church, as we wait we are to go and tell others what we have learned about Him. As you go, you tell someone and they tell someone and on and on the message of Jesus' saving power spreads throughout the world. We could be the generation that tells every people group, every nation, every tribe and every tongue about Jesus. But are we? Jesus is not going to be sent back until we do!

An evangelist came to preach a revival at our church. He told of what would happen if one person led another person to the LORD and those two people led two others to the LORD. Then it would be four and if those four people shared Christ with another four, then 16 would be saved, then 256, then 65536, then 4294967296, then 18446744073709551616 and so on. If we only would tell people about Jesus this could be the generation that reaches every people group to the LORD so Jesus can come back.

I have never been to First Step, but if you are in an abusive situation, if you are being beaten or raped or even if someone has left you, First Step may be the place you need to go first, or a family member's house or a friend's house. You need to get away from the person causing your pain. If you have been raped or molested, there is help to get over it, but first you have to get away from the one doing it to you.

Suicide is not the answer. God wants a living sacrifice— that means He needs you to be alive. He loves you too much for you to kill yourself. You can move past the pain of this moment in your life with Jesus' help. But sometimes we just need some people to be Jesus with skin on them. Trust Jesus but tell someone you need their help. Talk and keep talking until it is better.

Allowing someone else to drive for me right now helps until I get my medicines regulated and know how they affect me.

It helps to allow God to have complete control over my life. It is called surrender, but it took me a long time to do it. I pray because of this book your journey to surrender to Christ might be made easier and quicker than it was for me.

It is not easy to be bipolar. People tell me I have to hang in there. But it is not easy. It is not easy to be a Christian either. But I have never once regretted being one of God's own. God is love and love means meeting needs and that is what God does so well. But Abba does not spoil His children. God does not give us everything, nor should He. He meets our needs even deep needs nothing else can touch. He also gives us some of our wants and wishes too, but not all of them. God is wise; He knows what we can handle and what we cannot. Leave it in His hands about what to ask for: just ask Him.

Captivating by John and Stasi Eldredge based on pg 100

Prayer of my heart

Yes, Jesus, yes I do invite You in. Come to my heart in these shattered places. My heart broke into a million tiny little pieces during the days between when Buh left me for real and the weekend I became convinced that You, Jesus, came back — I thought the Rapture had happened and that I had been left behind. I was scared speechless. I have never been more afraid. My heart was devastated. And continuing on into the present every time when someone is in the room with me and suddenly without me knowing it, they move to another room, I would panic. Last year You started saying to me in my head or maybe to my heart, **"I will never leave you or forsake you."** Over and over You say it then You say, **"I will tell You that as many times as you need to hear it."** Thank You, I praise You. That has helped immeasurably. But I ask You, Jesus is there more healing You can do there. Come to me my Savior. I open this door of my heart. I give You permission to heal my wounds. Come to me here. Come for me here. Pour oil of Your Holy Spirit on my wounds. I plead the blood of Jesus on my sins, please forgive me. In Jesus Name, Amen.

One day Jesus is coming back to get His Bride the church—are we ready? Believers in Jesus, those who are in a relationship with Him, are the ones who will be taken up to be with Him forever. We will not all die; we shall be changed in a twinkling of an eye. Are you ready? There will be no time to make the decision when the rapture happens. You need to make that choice now.

Behold, I tell you a mystery: We shall not all sleep, but we shall all be changed—in a moment, in the twinkling of an eye, at the last trumpet. For the trumpet will sound, and the dead will be raised incorruptible, and we shall be changed. 1 Corinthians 15:51-52 (NKJV)

It does not matter even if we believe the rapture will happen. It will happen and if we are saved we can discuss it in the air with Jesus when it happens. Thank You Jesus that You are coming back for us some day. In that split second, life on earth will change dramatically. Christians who are taken will not be there to drive their cars and some of those cars will be on cruise control setting going 70 miles an hour with no one driving. Planes, trains and buses will wreck. There will be earthquakes, fire, famine, death and destruction. There will be something like locusts whose sting can torture for months the unbelievers. It is all foretold in the Bible. All other prophecies have come true from the Bible, these will too.

(45)

"Renounce the Agreements you've Made"

❧

*Y*our wounds brought messages with them, lots of messages. Somehow they all usually land in the same place. They had a similar theme. "It is your fault, Carol."
God spoke, **"Now Carol tell me what did it say to you when Buh left":**

> I do not please him.
> I do not do it right.
> I will never be able to make it on my own.
> I am not okay.
> I am not right..
> I am not a good mother to Jen and Jay.
> I am not a good wife.
> I am worthless.
> I am a disappointment.
> I am repulsive.
> I am too much…and not enough.

Jesus spoke, **"Now Carol tell me what did it say to you when you thought I left you?"**

> I was not good enough for You and never would be.
> I would never be saved.

I was all alone again.
Just asking for forgiveness was not enough.
None of my friends from church were there for me anymore.
I let You down.
I was wrong.

I started thinking how to survive without God and found I did not want to survive without God. God proved to me they were all the devil's lies. God taught me the truth of His Holy Bible and that He loves me.

Jesus, thank You that You have made everything all right. With You in my life I am complete in Christ. I do not have to worry about what it said to me after Buh left and after I thought Jesus left me behind. It was not true then and when You come back to get Your Bride the church, I am going with You. I praise God. In Jesus Name, Amen.

October Friday evening 10-3-08

Abba, thank You for answered prayer. Thank You, for new tears and new joys. I have started crying tears again. It helps to cry real tears. It feels good to cry again. I praise You, LORD. The tears rolled down my face and onto my hand. Thank You for You hold every tear in Your hands. I have had tears roll down my face when I was lying down, and they filled my ears. I have had them roll down my face and into my mouth, and I have tasted them. I have had tears collect on my glasses till I could hardly see straight. I will take the tears any day over not being able to cry. Thank You for the healing tears again.

God if You work with me tenderly, You can break my heart. Help me feel. Soften my heart; tender my heart, my tough heart, my hard heart. Circumcise my heart with the Sword of Your Spirit. Continue to show Yourself, God. Keep doing it even if I cry or even if it hurts. I pray for the filling and fruit of the Holy Spirit. Come Living Water and fill us to the brim, full to overflowing of Your Holy Spirit, into the empty places that are accidents waiting to happen. I pray Your Holy Spirit will bubble out the cracks You left in me on purpose.

You number my wanderings; Put my tears into Your bottle; Are they not in Your book? Psalm 56:8 (NKJV)

Abba, I pray to share the personality of Christ, and I ask in His Mighty Name, the Name of Christ, Amen.

That was a prayer of Beth Moore's from the Bible study, *To live is Christ the life and ministry of Paul.* I praise and thank God for how Beth Moore makes it easier to understand the Bible, and how it applies to me.

Abba, thank You for the Bible to live by and thank You for abundant life. I bless Your Name. LORD Jesus, teach me to pray. I praise You and I thank You. Teach me to walk in the Spirit. Teach me to pray in the Spirit, and teach me to dance in the Spirit to Your honor, praise and glory. In Jesus Name, Amen.

for prophecy never came by the will of man, but holy men of God spoke as they were moved by the Holy Spirit. 2 Peter 1:21 (NKJV)

Holy men of God wrote the scriptures so we can read it.

Dr. Snowden gave me two thumbs up for what I have been doing. I have been learning love languages. My Daddy's love language is service: I show my love for him by working for him. My Momma's love language is stuff and service. She feels loved when she is surrounded by things or people. There is a book I am supposed to read called *The Five Love Languages for Singles* by Gary Chapman. It explains that different people love differently. I did not understand their love language. I did not see what they were doing as showing their love for me. Learning this helped me show my love to Daddy by helping him burn some dead trees and the book helps me understand how they show me their actions are out of love for me.

October Saturday PM 10-4-08

Abba, Thank You. I do not have to go anywhere else to have some fun. Today Daddy, Bryan and I burned some trees. All the trees were dead except one live tree. Bryan cut them down earlier in the week. Daddy started four different fires with the largest logs and we kept adding all the other branches to each fire. I had fun. I even roasted some wieners on one of the logs of the fire. It was too hot to get up close, so I laid the wieners on a log that Bryan had moved out away from the fire to cook on. It was just coals and I left the wieners on the coals until they were kind of burned, just like I like them cooked. While I was breaking up the branches, I kept praying for You, Abba, to prune me and turn up the spiritual fire in me and let the dross come to the top and get rid of sin in me. I pray for 1,000 refinements at once. Let's start with forgiveness; there are still sins in me. I fall so short of Your glory and the standard You have set to live up to. Please forgive me.

Abba, I pray for Carolyn that everything goes well. I pray she comes to church Sunday to hear Michael, her son, give his testimony before he is ordained as a deacon. In Jesus Name, Amen.

October Monday 10-27-08

Abba, today I see Dr. Snowden, Bro. Randy and Pam all in the same day. What do we talk about? Please put a watch guard on my mouth that I will not say anything I am not supposed to say. Help me talk, but help me listen and write down what they say so I will not forget. I want to grow closer to You, LORD. Please let Jesus be the focus. You care about me. Thank You that You care about me. You love me by meeting my needs. I need Jesus. I desire Jesus. Please do not let me stray and sin against You. I pray for a peace that passes all understanding. In Jesus Name, Amen.

Dr. Snowden recommended I ask Dr. Wieck for some medicine to help the restless leg syndrome my medicine is causing. We talked about restoring my spirit. He used an example of two women:

One woman does task work; she does it because she has to. Example: cleaning, and picking dandelions.

Another woman does ministry work; she does it because she wants to. Example: cooking, writing, praying, quilting, the CD ministry, Faithbooking, teaching Sunday school and Vacation Bible School.

He explained that overload is giving away more than I get back, such as making work of a hobby which should be fun.

He talked about my being in the driver's seat and not hanging on to the back of the fire engine of life.

We talked about Jay and Melissa being close enough to visit and that I can invite them to come when it is convenient and go see them when I want to. I can talk to them and find a weekend good for both families.

Abba, Bro. Randy was busy this week. He went to go play golf with his Dad on his Dad's birthday. So Pam and I met together, just us girls. We did not really talk about anything important. We discussed what Dr. Snowden and I talked about. Mostly we just visited. She paid for a cherry limeade from Sonic for me and she got a diet Coke with vanilla, cherry and light on the ice. And we just talked. We talked about playing the Wii, about skating and the lake. It was nice not to have to think about important stuff and just relax and laugh awhile. In Jesus Name, Amen.

November Tuesday 11-11-08

Abba, yesterday I saw Bro. Randy and Pam for counseling. I have come a long way since I got bad around Spring break. I have improved greatly. I praise You for it. Thank You for the godly counsel You have placed in my life.

One of the things we talked about is my fear of being alone because of the time I had a manic episode where I believed I had been left behind. The wound is still fresh even after all these years. In Jesus Name, Amen.

Those left behind who take the mark of the beast will have no hope of ever being saved. Are you ready? Do not wait till then to choose Jesus. If you do not take the mark of the beast you will not be allowed to work or buy things. If you do take the mark of the beast you will never be able to be saved from that point on. There will be fire and famine, and death. Choose now, do not wait. It will be a difficult life after the rapture. God's full wrath will be poured out on the people of the earth. And there is no reason to wait. Trust Jesus now, today.

(46)

Everybody Needs to Have a Prayer Partner

December 12-12-09

I met Carolyn when a group from our church went Christmas caroling at her apartment two years ago. She was put on the CD ministry at our church, and I started visiting her. We became close friends immediately. We just hit it off right from the start. We can talk about anything together. I call her every night or she calls me and we pray together. We read a page from *Breaking Free Day by Day* by Beth Moore every night. Lately we sing together. Neither one of us sings very well but to God it is beautiful music to His ears. When we had to move out of the educational part of our church building to remodel, they were throwing away some old hymnals so I took a large print song book for me, one for Carolyn and one for JoBeth, her sister. We did not start singing right away. I do not even know how we began singing, but we sing a few songs at night before we pray.

Carolyn is bipolar, just like I am. We are a good match. She is a very special friend. She makes me laugh. This Christmas she helped me make presents for the three year olds I teach in Sunday school. We made beautiful barrette holders for the girls. We enjoy each other's company. We have been watching the love series movies based on Janet Oke's books. I do not watch much television, but the movies are so special.

When Carolyn and I pray, sometimes she prays first, sometimes I pray first and sometimes we pray together conversationally. I think our prayer time is the best part of the day. God listens and answers our prayers. It is as if He bends down from heaven and talks with us. It is a special time for both of us. The Bible says when two or three agree it is done in heaven.

"Again I say to you that if two of you agree on earth concerning anything that they ask, it will be done for them by My Father in heaven. For where two or three are gathered together in My name, I am there in the midst of them." Matthew 18:19-20 (NKJV)

If you are married, you could pray with your spouse. If you are not married, find a prayer partner; make a new friend if you have to. Find someone with whom you can learn to pray.

Carolyn and I pray about everything and everybody we can call to mind. We place it all into God's hands and pray His will be done. Knowing God is answering behind the scenes we go to sleep and rest peacefully. Prayer is talking and listening to God. It is like breathing in and out.

December Friday 12-18-09

Our prayer time is the best part of my day. It gets me ready for a sound sleep. We bring all our cares and worries and place them in God's capable hands and leave them there. Carolyn and I can talk about anything. We talk about the things that happened long ago or just today. And then we pray about it, trusting God to work His will. We pray He will answer in His will because His way is best, bigger and better than we can even think or imagine. He listens even when we do not have anything to say at the moment. He is so patient and kind. That is when He directs us as we pray; He reminds us of things about which we need to pray. Carolyn and I are learning all the Names of God and we are learning His characteristics, so we praise Him for who He is as well as what He does. We pray about anything and everything; nothing is too little or too big to pray about and ask for God's presence and God's help. Prayer is talking and listening. We listen to God's still small voice, and we listen by reading the Bible. God never asks us to do something contrary to His Word, the Bible. The Bible is our road map and instruction manual on how to live in this world. Christians do not belong to this world, our citizenship is in Heaven. We are ambassadors for Christ while we are here on earth. We are here for such a brief time, less than a fraction of a billi-second compared to how long we will be in Heaven with God. We seek God to see how we are to serve Him while we are still on this earth. Ask for God's wisdom, knowledge, understanding, revelation, sound judgment and discernment.

God loves to answer prayers when we ask with the right motive—to honor Him, praise Him and give Him the credit for answering our prayers. Sometimes God answers so big that we do not even recognize His answer as the answer to our prayers! Do not give up in your praying, sometimes it takes time. Ask God for patience in your prayers. And sometimes God answers before we voice it aloud. Sometimes God waits to see if we really want it. Sometimes God wants to personally get involved in the situation about which we have prayed. Sometimes God shows up big, sometimes He whispers. Sometimes God says "no," and that can be the best answer He can give.

God is not like us. We cannot comprehend, envision or imagine the Holiness of God. He is set apart from us. A chasm separates us from God and only Jesus' substitutionary death on the cross covers our sin and our shame. When we trust Christ to save us, the cross spans that chasm which exists between God and man. Then we can come to God the Father as Abba our DADDY. We become sons and daughters of God and joint heirs with Christ. When God saves us, Christ Jesus becomes our big Brother and our Husband to be. When we are saved, we pray for God to forgive us of our sins. We continue to sin, no one is perfect except Jesus. We still have to ask God on an ongoing basis how we have sinned against Him and agree with God in prayer to ask for forgiveness and repent of our sins.

If we confess our sins, He is faithful and just to forgive us our sins and to cleanse us from all unrighteousness. 1 John 1:9 (NKJV)

God sometimes answers our prayers quickly, and sometimes God does not answer in our life time. It is a relationship. There is nothing that you cannot talk (pray) about to God. Nothing is off limits. God already knows about it. God listens to our heart's cry even when we cannot put it into words. He listens, He loves, and He cares about the big and little of our prayers and about our daily existence. Jesus is fully God and fully man. He knows what it is like to live on this earth. He knows the heartaches and the losses. God became man and dwelt among us. Immanuel means "God with us. " Jesus can still be with us through His Holy Spirit. Each day put on the armor of God. We are not prepared for the day without Him. Ask to be filled with His Holy Spirit. Ask over and over again throughout the day.

Carolyn wrote this about our prayer time:

My prayer partner is the greatest gift God has given me. I think we both needed something or someone in our lives, and it turned out to be a best friend, a sister, a prayer partner, and someone who you can laugh with, cry with, watch movies with and most of all pray with. I look forward to my prayers we share every night. Sometimes I will start our prayers or she will start our prayers or we will both pray together. That is my favorite. God answers our prayers. We pray for everyone and everything and it is such a blessing to see our prayers answered. We both love God more than anything in this old world. He is our life. We live to love Him. I have always prayed and had special time for God and His Word. I just did not know a prayer partner could answer your needs in such a special way. When we pray, God is right beside us. I am sure we make Him smile and cry at times. You see God handpicked us, put us together to do things pleasing unto Him. We even sing together, we both got old hymnals at church when they were getting rid of them. So we now have our own song books. We usually sing about three songs each night, and if you ever heard me sing, you would know why I said God smiles on us. I am closer to God than I have ever been. I will always believe having a prayer partner changed my life. I have the very best prayer partner in the world. I think everyone needs a prayer partner. I truly believe it is a life changing thing. When I met Carol, she hardly ever smiled. I can make her laugh, Glory to God, because she needed to laugh and smile. She is such a beautiful person, and she will never know how much I love her, and how my life has changed, thanks to her. She has taught me a lot about God. She is such a wonderful Christian. I wish I was half the Christian that she is. She is a real blessing to me and I thank God for my very special friend each and every day.

(47)

Though your Sins be as Scarlet

February 2-11-10 Thursday

*I*t is snowing outside this morning. It started sometime after 5:00 AM. I woke up at 7:30 AM and the ground is already covered. It is so beautiful. I walked to the mailbox and listened to the scrunch of my footsteps in the snow. The snow reminds me that though my sins be as scarlet they shall be as white as snow because of Jesus death on the cross. There is forgiveness of sin because of the blood Jesus shed at the cross. Do you trust Jesus, He is so trustworthy.

I went to see Dr. Snowden on Tuesday. I needed to talk to him. I started having panic attacks again. When I told Dr. Wieck a few weeks ago, he increased my medicine. But I wanted to know why I was having them. Dr. Snowden knows the right questions to ask. I told Dr. Snowden that I have tried suicide when I had panic attacks in the past. Suicide is a permanent solution to a temporary problem. I do not like having panic attacks. But I do not get scared as I did when they first started years ago. I guess I pray my way through the panic attacks now. I am not afraid of them anymore. I breathe in and breathe out, in through the nose and out through the mouth. And when I breathe I use my abdomen instead of my chest; it is called my diaphragm. If you use your chest, it is too shallow of a breath. Calm down, relax and it will subside. The panic attacks subside if I do my breathing exercises, Dr. Snowden taught me how to relax that way. And while you do that, pray the same way, breathe in and breathe out. Lift a prayer up to God and listen for His still small voice, in and out.

If you confess to God your sins, He is faithful and true to forgive your sins. I want to ask forgiveness so soon that when the devil tells on me to God, it is all ready forgiven and God responds, "**What sin**?"

(48)

How Can you Know
Jesus Loves you?

Jesus is speaking:

> "A little while longer and the world will see Me no more, but you will see Me. Because I live, you will live also. At that day you will know that I am in My Father, and you in Me, and I in you. He who has My commandments and keeps them, it is he who loves Me. And he who loves Me will be loved by My Father, and I will love him and manifest Myself to him." John 14:19-21 (NKJV)

"Jesus loves me, this I know for the Bible tells me so," is a little song, but so true.

Jesus loves me

By Anna B. Warner

Jesus loves me! this I know, For the Bible tells me so; Little ones to Him belong; They are weak, but He is strong.

Jesus loves me! He who died Heaven's gates to open wide! He will wash away my sin; Let His little child come in.

Jesus loves me! Loves me still, Tho I am very weak and ill; From His shining throne on high, comes to watch me where I lie.

Jesus loves me! He will stay close beside me all the way; If I love Him, when I die He will take me home on high.

Yes, Jesus loves me, Yes, Jesus loves me, Yes, Jesus loves me, The Bible tells me so.

*H*ow do I know Jesus loves me? God talks to me in a still, small voice and through the Bible. He talks to me about little and big things, important things and not so important things. God is teaching me to recognize His voice as opposed to Satan's voice or one of his demons, but God is also helping me to recognize my own voice. I need to learn to recognize God's voice and listen and obey only His voice and not to all the other voices going on in my head.

If you are alone in this world, it is good to have Jesus as your friend. He wants to be your Best Friend. The Holy Spirit is Counselor and Comforter and Helper. Ask God to fill you with His Holy Spirit and He will, day by day keep asking to be filled by God's Holy Spirit. God answers prayer exceedingly, abundantly above what we ask or think.

Now to Him who is able to do exceedingly abundantly above all that we ask or think, according to the power that works in us, to Him be glory in the church by Christ Jesus to all generations, forever and ever. Amen. Ephesians 3:20-21 (NKJV)

Watch and see how God answers your prayers. God answers big so sometime we have trouble seeing His answer as the answer to our prayers. God always answers prayer, and sometimes no is the very best answer He can give us. It is for our best interest, so when we pray we should always ask for God's will to be done. God only says no so He can give us a bigger and better yes. Keep a journal and record how God answers your prayers. If we do not write them down, we tend to forget even asking Him. Thank Him and praise Him for His answers.

Read God's Word, the Holy Bible, and pray before you study the Bible for godly wisdom, understanding, knowledge, revelation, sound judgment and discernment. God never tires of answering that prayer. I believe God loves to hear the pages turning in our Bibles. It is God's love letter to us, unless you are not being obedient and then it can be God's convicting. Ask God to forgive you and He will. Repent and turn away from your sin, He can and will help you get past your sin. He does not expect you to do it alone. He wants to help you turn away from your sin. Jesus sees all you do right. He forgives, as you ask Him, all you do wrong against Him. There is now no condemnation for those who are in Christ Jesus.

There is therefore now no condemnation to those who are in Christ Jesus, who do not walk according to the flesh, but according to the Spirit. Romans 8:1 (NKJV)

For God did not send His Son into the world to con-demn the world, but that the world through Him might be saved. John 3:17 (NKJV)

It really does not matter if you believe in heaven or hell; one of those places is where you will spend eternity. Choose Jesus and you gain heaven. Reject Jesus and you lose and your eternity will be hell forever. It is no game. God does not play games. The choice is yours to make. Choose Jesus and choose wisely. Ask God to forgive your sins based on Jesus Christ's death on the cross where He paid for your sins by His own blood. Do not let Jesus' death on the cross count for nothing in your life. Jesus died for you because He loves you so much He would rather die than live without you. Do not put off your decision for another day to trust Jesus to save you. Do not try to put off your decision until you straighten up your life. God can handle your sin problems. Jesus' blood is what cleanses our sins. God can help you with your sins once you come into a relationship with Jesus Christ. Trust Him. He forgave my sins. He can forgive yours. God is patiently waiting for you. Do you want forgiveness? Just ask for forgiveness in Jesus Name.

Jesus is the only one who makes me good enough for God. It is not what I do, it is what Jesus did when He paid my sin penalty on the cross. And then three days later He came back alive to prove to everyone that He was God.

Jesus saves even me as bad as I was, even you no matter what you have done. Trust Him, He will hold you in His arms and forgive you if you will only ask for forgiveness. Jesus can forgive any sin except for not believing in Him.

Forgive me LORD God. Hold me in Your arms, LORD Jesus. Thank You and I praise You. I was never alone. Jesus was with me all the time only I could not understand it then. I just could not see it.

Asking for forgiveness and turning from your sins and to Jesus is the most important thing you can do in this life. Ask Jesus into your heart and life. Jesus came into my heart and life and into all the broken places.

When Bro. Donald came to our church and preached a revival, he gave as an illustration: the parable of the car. "He had an ugly car, as ugly as sin," he said. The service lights came on. He weighed his options—go on or turn back. He decided to go to a mechanic. He took his car to the shop. It could have been the coolant because the temperature sensor was on. It could have been the oil because the oil pressure light was on. It could have been the gas and he might not have had enough gas to get to his destination.

He gave the mechanic permission to fix the car. When God made Adam and Eve, they were in tune with God then they sinned and the wages of sin is death.

For the wages of sin is death, but the gift of God is eternal life in Christ Jesus our Lord. Roman 6:23 (NKJV)

Pray and say, "Jesus, fix my sin problem." Only Jesus can fix your sin problem. Jesus lived a sinless life that means He never sinned, not one time. Therefore when He died on the cross, for our sins, He was the perfect sacrifice. Jesus paid the sin penalty for our sins. Jesus died on the cross for you and me—for all, who will trust Him. Jesus arose from the dead three days later in victory!

Bro. Donald had to pay to get his car fixed. Though the wages of sin is death, Jesus can fix our sin problem.

"Come now, and let us reason together," Says the LORD, "Though your sins are like scarlet, They shall be as white as snow; Though they are red like crimson, They shall be as wool. Isaiah 1:18 (NKJV)

As far as the east is from the west, So far has He removed our transgressions from us. Psalm 103:12 (NKJV)

Bro. Donald took a small piece of paper which represented our sin. And he lit the paper. Jesus represented the lighter and what He does with our sin. The paper never fell to the ground it burned so fast. Jesus completely forgives. Jesus does not make us better, He makes us new.

Pray and ask God to examine your heart. Trust Jesus and give Him permission to take your sin away. Pray and talk to God:

Dear Jesus, thank You for dying for my sin. I realize I am a sinner and that I am separated from You. But right this minute I confess my sin to You. Please forgive me and take away my sin. Change my life and I give You permission to have complete control of my life. Come into my heart today. I ask in Jesus Name, Amen.

Now you too have a positive testimony to tell about how Jesus saved you just now. You have a lifetime ahead of you to tell people how Jesus will continue to save you daily. Tell someone today about how you were saved.

(49)

When Temptation Becomes Sin

ဥ

*C*indy was the one who taught me that just because I am tempted; it does not mean I sin. It is only when I act on the temptation by thinking about it, or talking about it, or doing it that it becomes a sin.

> Let no one say when he is tempted, "I am tempted by God"; for God cannot be tempted by evil, nor does He Himself tempt anyone. But each one is tempted when he is drawn away by his own desires and enticed. Then, when desire has conceived, it gives birth to sin; and sin, when it is full-grown, brings forth death. James 1:13-15 (NKJV)

From *the Billy Graham Training Center Bible* notes:
Temptation—God does not tempt

God is holy and has no inclination toward evil. He is not the author of sin, nor is He responsible for sin's entrance into the human race. God is permitting evil to run its course until His plan of redemption reaches its culmination. God cannot be tempted, nor does He tempt anyone. Though He allows us to be tempted, God has placed limits on Satan's activities and the extent of his power to tempt us. God is always in control.

Though it might seem so, evil does not reign unbridled on the earth. In the true story of Job, Satan reports in to God and discusses Job in order to obtain permission to tempt him.

Now there was a day when the sons of God came to present themselves before the LORD, and Satan also came among them. And the LORD said to Satan, "From where do you come?" So Satan answered the LORD and said, "From going to and fro on the earth, and from walking back and forth on it." Then the LORD said to Satan, "Have you considered My servant Job, that there is none like him on the earth, a blameless and upright man, one who fears God and shuns evil?" So Satan answered the LORD and said, "Does Job fear God for nothing? Have You not made a hedge around him, around his household, all that he has on every side? You have blessed the work of his hands, and his possessions have increased in the land. But now, stretch out Your hand and touch all that he has, and he will surely curse You to Your face!" And the LORD said to Satan, "Behold, all that he has is in your power; only do not lay a hand on his person." So Satan went out from the presence of the LORD. Job 1:6-12 (NKJV)

Job lost his property, all his oxen, donkeys, sheep, camels, all his children and all his servants, except the four servants who brought him the bad news, he lost seven sons and three daughters but his wife was still alive.

Then Job arose, tore his robe, and shaved his head; and he fell to the ground and worshiped. And he said: "Naked I came from my mother's womb, And naked shall I return there. The LORD gave, and the LORD has taken away; Blessed be the name of the LORD." Job 1:20-22 (NKJV)

Again there was a day when the sons of God came to present themselves before the LORD, and Satan came also among them to present himself before the LORD. And the LORD said to Satan, "From where do you come? Satan answered the LORD and said, "From going to and fro on the earth, and from walking back and forth on it." Then the LORD said to Satan, "Have you considered My servant Job, that there is none like him on the earth, a blameless and upright man, one who fears God and shuns evil? And still he holds fast to his integrity, although you incited Me against him, to destroy him without cause." So Satan answered the LORD and said, "Skin for skin! Yes all that a man has he will give for his life. But stretch out Your hand now, and touch his bone and his flesh, and he will surely curse You to Your face!" And the LORD said to Satan, "Behold he is in your hand, but spare his life." So Satan went out from the presence of the LORD, and struck Job with painful boils from the sole of his foot to the crown of his head. And he took for himself a potsherd with which to scrape himself while he sat in the midst of the ashes. Then his wife said to him, "Do you still hold fast to your integrity? Curse God and die!" But he said to her, "You speak as one of the foolish women speaks. Shall we indeed accept good from God, and shall we not accept adversity? In all this Job did not sin with his lips. Job 2:1-10 (NKJV)

Again from *the Billy Graham Training Center Bible* notes: Temptation—God does not tempt.

God permitted Satan to subject Job to a severe, though limited, temptation. God sustained Job through the trial, and gave him far more than Job had lost.

Even Jesus was tempted yet without sin.

> *For we do not have a High Priest who cannot sympathize with our weaknesses, but was in all points tempted as we are, yet without sin.* Hebrews 4:15 (NKJV)

Do not try to clean yourself up before you come to Christ for salvation. We come to Christ first and God forgives us of all our sin. He starts gently to clean us up. He starts changing the "want to" in us. Jesus gives us the desire to not sin, but to obey Him. But you have to come to Him and be saved first. Then Jesus empowers us to live the Christ life. The Christ life is beyond your wildest expectations or imaginations—beyond your hopes and dreams. Jesus is past understanding. When you ask to be filled with His Holy Spirit; He will overflow you with His fullness. Do not be afraid of the Holy Spirit.

> *For unto us a Child is born, Unto us a Son is given; And the government will be upon His shoulder. And His name will be called Wonderful, Counselor, Mighty God, Everlasting Father, Prince of Peace.* Isaiah 9:6 (NKJV)

Jesus is speaking:

> *"If you love Me, keep My commandments. And I will pray the Father, and He will give you another Helper, that He may abide with you forever—the Spirit of truth, whom the world cannot receive, because it neither sees Him nor knows Him, but you know Him, for He dwells with you and will be in you. I will not leave you orphans; I will come to you.* John 14:15-18 (NKJV)

> *But the Helper, the Holy Spirit, whom the Father will send in My name, He will teach you all things, and bring to your remembrance all things that I said to you.* John 14:26 (NKJV)

Jesus tells us:

> *Nevertheless I tell you the truth. It is to your advantage that I go away; for if I do not go away, the Helper will not come to you; but if I depart, I will send Him to you. And when He has come, He will convict the world of sin, and of righteousness, and of judgment: of sin, because they do not believe in Me; of righteousness, because I go to My Father and you see Me no more; of judgment, because the ruler of this world is judged. "I still have many things to say to you, but you cannot bear them now. However, when He, the Spirit of truth, has come, He will guide you into all truth; for He will not speak on His own authority, but whatever He hears He will speak; and He will tell you things to come. He will glorify Me, for He will take of what is Mine and declare it to you. All things that the Father has are Mine. Therefore I said that He will take of Mine and declare it to you. "A little while, and you will not see Me; and again a little while, and you will see Me, because I go to the Father.* John 16:7-16 (NKJV)

The Holy Spirit is Counselor, Comforter and the Helper. He leads and guides us. He interprets our prayers and presents them perfectly to our Abba Father. The Holy Spirit helps us pray and when we do not think we can, He will pray for us.

> *Likewise the Spirit also helps in our weaknesses. For we do not know what we should pray for as we ought, but the Spirit Himself makes intercession for us with groaning which cannot be uttered. Now He who searches the hearts knows what the mind of the Spirit is, because He makes intercession for the saints according to the will of God.* Romans 8:26-27 (NKJV)

The Holy Spirit dispels the fears in us, He gives us faith and strength until encouragement is the end product. God wants us to be courageous enough to share Christ with the lost people around us. The Bible tells us that Jesus is delaying His coming again because He is not willing that any should perish.

> *The Lord is not slack concerning His promise, as some count slackness, but is longsuffering toward us, not willing that any should perish but that all should come to repentance.* 2 Peter 3:9 (NKJV)

There are still millions and millions in different people groups around the world who have never even heard the name Jesus much less of His saving grace. There is no plan B, we are it. It is up to us to tell people about Jesus. We can pray, we can go, we can give, or we can do all three. As you go: tell the story of how you came to Christ; tell the stories you know from the Bible, share God's Word.

> *And Jesus came and spoke to them, saying, "All authority has been given to Me in heaven and on earth. Go therefore and make disciples of all the nations, baptizing them in the name of the Father and of the Son and of the Holy Spirit, teaching them to observe all things that I have commanded you; and lo, I am with you always, even to the end of the age." Amen.* Matthew 28:18-20 (NKJV)

Jesus can meet your needs. Most especially deep needs no one else has been able to reach or to touch. He will not do it unless you ask Him. He is a gentleman. He will not barge in on your life, but when asked, He can make all the difference in the world in your life and in those around you.

Meeting needs is Jesus Christ's specialty that is how He shows us His love. Come to Him today. He is waiting just for you. Beth Moore said in the *Breaking Free* devotional that we think Heaven will be Heaven because God will be there but God thinks Heaven will be Heaven because we will be there.

For there is one God and one Mediator between God and men, the Man Christ Jesus, who gave Himself a ransom for all, to be testified in due time, 1 Timothy 2:5-6 (NKJV)

Abba, You never left me. Thank You and I praise You. You never will leave me. Thank You and I praise You. Thank You for saving me when You did. Just in time. You are never early or late. You are always just in the nick of time. My Knight in shining armor, You are King of kings and LORD of lords. You came to rescue me before…before I was born or even thought of…before the manic depression…before I realized how much I needed You… before I needed a Savior… before I needed You as my Husband …before I needed You as my very Best Friend…before I needed You as my Counselor… before the divorce…before I knew I could live forever with You and that eternity starts the very moment we ask Jesus into our hearts and lives…before I knew I could be a new creation in Christ…before I knew that the old things pass away behold all things are new. You came to me just in time.

Thank You just does not sound like enough—but I thank You. I praise You. I worship You. I honor You. I hold You in high esteem. I am in awe of You. I am so proud of You. You are my Rock, my firm foundation. Forgive me I fail You so miserably. Help me. I need to be a woman after Your own heart. I need to walk with You, Jesus through every day—through all eternity. I am sorry I fall so short of Your glory, forgive me. I respect You Jesus. One day in heaven we will marry at the marriage supper of the Lamb. You covenanted with me to marry me, and Jesus has gone to prepare a place for me. The Holy Spirit is Your seal of promise. Thank You and I praise You. You love me and love means meeting needs. You, my love, meet my needs. Help me to tell others about what a great God You are. I pray to love You in return and I pray others will know how much I love You by how much I love them. God, my God, my Three in One, the Trinity, help me. Help me bloom where You plant me and shine Jesus shine through the cracks of this broken vessel as You put me back together. All the glory goes to You, my Abba Father, Jesus my Savior and Rescuer and Your Holy Spirit. I ask in the Name above all names, the Name of Jesus, Amen.

(50)

The First Sermon
I Heard Bro. Randy Preach

*I*t helped me know how I should live my life and why I should do the things I do.

Sunday, December 31, 2006.

We can experience God in a great way through our need, lack and insufficiency. How do we get Christ emanating through our pores, so people see Christ coming from our lips. If we really want to live the Christ life—Jesus was rejected and martyred by men, he was persecuted greatly, and maligned by religious leaders—we can expect no less.

Bro. Randy's prayer to begin this message was something like this:
"I need less of me and more of You, Jesus.
I need a mature faith in You.
I need Your Holy Spirit to fill me.
I need You to live in me.
I need to serve You.
I need to have a passion for You.

Not just on Sundays and Wednesdays or when I am only around other Christians but with everyone I encounter I need the Christ's life to show through me."

Paul said:

For to me, to live is Christ, and to die is gain. Philippians 1:21 (NKJV)

The Christ life is extremely costly. Serve Christ, even if no one listens to you. Be properly motivated. Do not do it for pay, nor because Bro. Ricky or Bro. Bill or Bro. Ted or Bro. Randy says you should. Know why you are doing what you are doing. Bro. Randy also prayed:

Father God, as we come before Your Holy Word we pray that it would come alive and active and sharp and that it would pierce deep within our hearts, that we might know if we are living religiosity for our own comfort and ease or whether in fact we are forging ahead to serve You no matter what the cost. And so Father just as You motivated Isaiah so too may You motivate us. May we learn from You this morning. I pray may Your grace be upon us. In Christ's Name, Amen.

The first point of the sermon was: know why you are doing what you are doing.

In the year that King Uzziah died, I saw the Lord sitting on a throne, high and lifted up, and the train of His robe filled the temple. Above it stood seraphim; each one had six wings: with two he covered his face, with two he covered his feet, and with two he flew. And one cried to another and said: "Holy, holy, holy is the LORD of hosts; The whole earth is full of His glory!" And the posts of the door were shaken by the voice of him who cried out, and the house was filled with smoke. Isaiah 6:1-4 (NKJV)

Foremost see the glory of God. It has to be for the Glory of God. The proper motivation: understand who God is—to go into the teeth of the devil and hell itself. It was not a vision or dream. Isaiah went into the temple in heaven. Isaiah knew King Uzziah—He only thought he had seen majesty. God opened his eyes to the glory of the LORD.

These things Jesus spoke, and departed, and was hidden from them. But although He had done so many signs before them, they did not believe in Him, that the word of Isaiah the prophet might be fulfilled, which he spoke: "Lord, who has believed our report? And to whom has the arm of the LORD been revealed?" Therefore they could not believe, because Isaiah said again: "He has blinded their eyes and hardened their hearts, Lest they should see with their eyes, Lest they should understand with their hearts and turn, So that I should heal them." These things Isaiah said when he saw His glory and spoke of Him. John 12:36B-41 (NKJV)

Spoke of whom? Jesus Christ. The eternal King of kings and LORD of lords, seated on the throne, 739 years before Jesus was born in the flesh in Bethlehem, this one who is eternally the King and sometimes during the Christmas season we picture Him in the manger and that is good, but we tend to leave Him there and think of Him as helpless and pitiful. He has always been King of kings; He will always be King of kings. He emptied Himself or divested Himself of some of the prerogatives of His deity for a short time to descend to this cruel estate to be a sacrifice for you and I but He is eternally Alpha and Omega, He has always been the King and He has always been on His throne and Isaiah was seeing none other than Jesus Christ Himself on the throne 700 and something years before He was born on earth.

Oh, and let me tell you what, it filled Isaiah's mind. He needed to get a big view of his Savior whom he was going to tell about and he was getting a big view of his Savior. Look at the things that are going on here. Seraphim, angelic beings, are above Him. Listen, Isaiah is in the temple and in the Holy of Holies which was to the Jew considered a place where only one person went once a year and that is the High Priest and yet he is there in vision and he is not just seeing the ark of the covenant and he is not just seeing the smoke of incense rise and he is not just seeing carved angels above the ark of the covenant. Isaiah is seeing a living situation going on in the throne room of heaven. He is seeing these live angelic creatures who have six wings and hands and feet and they obviously speak a human language because in a minute they say, "Holy, holy, holy is the LORD of hosts; the whole earth is full of His glory!" They are attending the King of kings, but the interesting thing is; it says with these three pairs of wings, only two of them are used to fly, and serve and attend the King of kings. With two of them they cover their face, because the majesty of this situation is so incomprehensible that even holy angelic beings cannot even look upon the King of kings. God allowed Moses to only see His backside as He passed by, yet Moses came down beamin' for days. This glory of which Isaiah spoke was so magnificent that these angelic beings have to use two of their wings to cover their face. And it is such an humbling thing for them that their feet, which are the most ignoble part of their anatomy, are covered with the other two pair of wings as if to say we do not deserve to even be in here, I want you to see what it was that they wanted to ring in the mind and in the heart of the one who was going to go out and serve. What they needed to know and what you and I need to know was what they said as they cried out to one another in an antiphonal recanting. It says in Isaiah 6:3: "One called out to another and said: Holy, holy, holy is the LORD of Hosts and the whole earth is full of His glory." In Hebrew the word for holy is "quadosh" Do you know what it means? It means cut off, it means chopped off. Do you know why it means that? Because God wants us to realize that He is God and we are not. This is where it has to start. And we do not even deserve to come in

His presence. He is cut off from us, completely and totally in His Holiness. And whatever filthy, little, righteous deeds that you do, that you think you can bring before God to bridge the chasm that exists between you and He, is not doodley squat. In fact the word of God says that it is filthy rags. Your righteous deeds are filthy rags before Holy God.

Let me tell you what happens as we live out our days, come to church and what not. We all tend to measure our righteousness and our holiness by looking' at each other. We think, "I am a little better than so and so." That is a relative holiness. Let me tell you something God wanted to snap Isaiah out of that mess. Isaiah's a "big dog" prophet; he is probably as holy a guy as there is in all of Jerusalem. Yet God wants to let him know right up front and without any question that he is absolutely cut off from Holy God. The chasm is so great that it is humanly unbridgeable.

How is God going to prepare His servant? He needs to see God's glory. He needs to recapture who God is. He needs to know that God is holy God, and a majestic God. The train of His robe fills the temple and angelic beings constantly praise and adore Him and smoke rises up and the thresholds tremble like an earthquake. God shows him this scene. God knows He is going to call him to a hard ministry path. Nobody is going to listen, nobody is going to care, nobody is going to follow, and they are going to turn away from God.

Now we live in a day and time when there are a whole lot of special effects and things like that but I am sure this got Isaiah's attention. I guarantee it would get ours as well. You say, "Well, I have not ever had that experience, so how can I be prepared to start living 2007 to the glory of God and getting constantly beaten, pushed down, maligned and rejected as I live the Christ's life. As sure as we sit here right now, we might not see it with physical eyes but with eyes of faith we know that it is going on right now! The Word of God tells us. And we believe it because we do not see with physical eyes. The King of Kings is on His throne. And the angelic creatures are worshiping Him and the threshold is shaking and quaking and they are crying: Holy, holy, holy to the character of the LORD Jesus Christ and so it applies to us just like it did to Isaiah. So what did Isaiah do? The first words that came out of his mouth and I have a feeling it took awhile. The first words that came out of his mouth and this is what he says:

So I said:"Woe is me, for I am undone! Because I am a man of unclean lips, And I dwell in the midst of a people of unclean lips; For my eyes have seen the King, The LORD of hosts." Isaiah 6:5 (NKJV) (Undone means ruined)

There is not any stronger word than the word woe! It means it is over for me. It means I am done, I am finished, and it is over. Knocked him on his face! And I bet you that if he could have dug and clawed and scratched and got under the ground he would have done it. Because he began to understand the chasm that exists between Holy God and unholy Isaiah (and unholy us) And so Isaiah is not coming and saying. "God I have done this for you and done that, and I am the top prophet. I talked to King Uzziah." I imagine he groveled; he would have done anything to get out of there. "Woe is me I am finished"

The Bible tells us the wages of sin is death. It is true. He knew it and he felt it deep within his soul as he stood before Holy King Jesus. God begins to prepare this man to go out. The first thing God does is to say, "I want you to recapture My glory. You have to see who I am! You have to know who I am! If you are going to be able to face the difficulties you have got to see, that I am majestic, Holy King Jesus!" What follows from that is that Isaiah begins to have an incredible sense of his own guilt before King Jesus. "Woe is me." "I am undone." "I am finished." Isaiah was not looking at how righteous he was or looking at what he had done or that he had been a prophet all these years. I think it is imperative for you and I, as well, to recapture the vision of our God by interacting with His Word and seeing, through eyes of faith, the truth of what is going on, to see who He is, how awesome He is, all that He does for us and to see His majesty. As we begin to do that it ought to humble us completely and knock us flat on our face.

What happens next is the real victory. God does not leave him on his face crying out. God wanted him to realize who he was before Holy God. Look at what happens.

> *Then one of the seraphim flew to me, having in his hand a live coal which he had taken with the tongs from the altar. And he touched my mouth with it, and said: "Behold, this has touched your lips; your iniquity is taken away, And your sin purged."* Isaiah 6:6-7 (NKJV) (Purged means forgiven).

You see: He saw the glory of God! He felt his guilt before God! He experienced the amazing grace of God! God wanted him to know that there was not a thing in the world that Isaiah could do. The angelic creature, by God's command no doubt, went to the alter and removed a hot, flaming, burning coal to apply to Isaiah's lips. Holy beings were crying "Holy, holy, holy", he could not even say things like that "I am a man of unclean lips." All that is within my heart comes out of my mouth and I know who I am. What God did through that angelic being is he took tongs with a hot coal from the altar of sacrifice on which Christ died and he touched his lips and removed his iniquity. It is all God. It is called grace. It is all God. It is all God!

And so this man who might have thought himself of high position, "I am the preacher boy, I am the prophet, and I go to King Uzziah and I go do all of these other things. Isaiah is not thinking that any more. He's thinking, God is glorious and I am insurmountably separated from Him. But for whatever, reason, in His grace, He has removed that which separates me from Him which is namely my unholiness and He has restored me to Himself!

John Newton had a somewhat similar experience in the 18th century. That old raunchy, seafaring man who was a slave trader and lived a hellatious lifestyle. By God's grace he was saved one night when he was out on stormy seas. He got out on the bow of that ship and then wrote the song, Amazing Grace.

"Amazing Grace, how sweet the sound that saved a wretch like me, I once was lost but now I am found. I was blind but now I see. Twas grace that taught my heart first of all to fear this Holy God and then it was also grace that my fears relieved. How precious did it first appear the hour that I first believed."

Listen, if you are going to have the motivation to go out and get chopped down and get made fun of and maybe even martyred for the cause of living the Christ life. You better understand GRACE!

It begins with glory. It begins with your guilt. And then you did not do anything to get to God, God did everything to get to you. That is called grace.

Do you know the reason Isaiah served God the rest of his life as he arose every day?

Isaiah saw the glory, he felt the guilt, he experienced the grace and he responded the only way we should respond, with gratitude. It is called gratitude. "Thank You God!" Isaiah said:

Also I heard the voice of the Lord, saying: "Whom shall I send, And who will go for Us?"

Then I said, "Here am I! Send me." Isaiah 6:8 (NKJV)

Isaiah was like a kid in kindergarten, with hand raised high and waving:
Please let me go!
Please let me go!
Please let me go!
But You are going to get shot down.
Please let me go!
But You are going to be made fun of.
Please, here I am!
Let me go!
Let me volunteer.

You are going to be maligned. You may even be martyred.
(Said with the same determination but perhaps softer and quieter) Please let me go!
The only proper motivation for living the Christ life is gratitude.

You are so deeply moved by and at what God has done to redeem your soul from condemnation through His Precious Son Jesus that you say, please let me go!

And if they make fun of me at school, or that hateful neighbor is mean to me or whatever happens to me, I will get up the next morning, it is tough, I do not like it, but I will keep going because of what God has done for me!

Father, as we begin 2007 and we consider the challenges of living for Christ in an ever increasing God-less society where we are aliens and strangers, we need a fresh motivation. It does not need to be Bro. Ricky up here telling us we need to do this or we need to do that. It does not need to be Bro. Randy telling us we need to do this or that. It does not need to be guilt. It does not need to be religiosity. It needs to be gratitude! No one ought to have to tell us to do anything when we've seen the glory of God and felt our guilt and experienced His amazing grace. No one ought to tell us to do anything. We ought to be sitting in the "classroom" with our hands, sticking in the air saying:

Please, please, please, please God use me!
So Father, I would just ask, that You would do that very thing in me. In Jesus Name, Amen.

*****

Charles Stanley's example as Bro. Randy explained it: God envelopes us Christians with a shield—a protective covering—and nothing, absolutely nothing, gets in to us except it is allowed by God. And, God can not only handle anything He lets through—He can use it for His glory, and if He cannot then He can take me home to be with Him in glory! This is Jesus' kingdom—it all belongs to Him.

(51)

How to Pray When you are Troubled

S ome sermons stand out to me more than others. This one
has become a part of my prayers since the first time I
heard it on March 4, 2008. Bro. Randy preached it on a Sunday
night at church and it has become a daily prayer for me since
that time. The following is based on his sermon that night. He
was kind enough to allow me to use his sermon notes but this
is also based on what I have learned by praying it daily since I
heard the sermon and studying Psalm 119 on my own.

The special music that Sunday night was by Diane. The
song she sang was written by Gorden Jenson: "I love you, I
love you, that's what Calvary said, I love you, I love you, I love
you written in red."

Some Bibles have just the words of Jesus written in red
printing. All the words in the Bible are written in red, not just
Jesus' words, but all of them. The Old Testament looks forward to Calvary. The New Testament looks back to Calvary. It
is all written in red.

What is the typical prayer request uttered from the lips
of those who are suffering? "Why? Why is this happening
to me?" And "Get me out of this! While these are the typical
prayer request—even from most Christians—they are not the

spiritually-mature requests. Spiritually-mature requests reflect a restful dependence on God, that He is in control and He is going to do what is best. That is why Peter urged,

Therefore, let those who suffer according to the will of God commit their souls to Him in doing good, as to a faithful Creator. I Peter 4:19 (NKJV)

The writer of Psalm 119—although living 1,000 years prior to Peter's exhortation—fulfilled the spirit of this verse to a "t." He definitely suffered, he suffered according to the will of God; he entrusted himself to his Creator, and he continued to do what was right. As such, he serves as a model of biblical response to those who suffer persecution.

Bro. Randy gave examples of some of the people who are in our church and people where he worked as a hospice chaplain before coming here to be our pastor. He mentioned people who suffered greatly, yet remained true and faithful to Christ. I wanted to share Sandra's story with you, so I called her and she shared her story with me to put into the book.

Sandra is the sweetest lady you will ever meet. Her husband, Bro. Jim, is our minister of music, and they always have a smile on their faces. Bro. Jim takes good care of Sandra, who has multiple sclerosis and is confined to a wheelchair at home. She dearly loves coming to church, but now sometimes she cannot come. She has a ministry of sharing what God has done in her life in spite of the disease that has caused her to be unable to walk. Her prayer ministry and her testimony is something she shares with us. She did not always accept her disease. At first she was very depressed and cried a lot because she was only given six to ten years to live. Sandra was 23 at the time with a husband and two small children at home.

Betty Moon went to see Sandra. Betty told her, with Bible in hand and trembling, "I just have to come to talk to you because I saw a black cloud hovering over your house. I felt like we needed to have prayer." Betty asked Sandra if she minded if she led in the prayer and Sandra told her she did not mind. Betty prayed one of the most gracious prayers Sandra had ever heard. "Do not question any of this. You just rely upon the LORD. We are going to remember you in prayer. With all the prayers going up, the LORD hears them."

Sandra left it in God's hands. Little things started happening, and they were for the good. People asked her to give her testimony at different churches. At 71 years of age Sandra is still going strong. And she praises the LORD for it, and she still can hardly believe it. She praises God because she knows He is responsible for her still being alive.

Now for the background of the sermon Bro. Randy preached. Most Bible scholars believe the writer of Psalm 119 to be either David or Daniel. For our purposes, it matters not which one.

Both men suffered, suffered greatly and for long periods of time. In their suffering they turned to God. And as such, serve as models of mature response to all of us who face trials, tests, and tribulation in our lives.

David was a man after God's own heart. He wrote many of the Psalms from his heart. David knows suffering and trouble. You have, or will have trials, sufferings and troubles. We are just shovels, rakes, picks and hoes, unless the Master picks us up and uses us—we are nothing.

Your hands have made me and fashioned me; Give me understanding, that I may learn Your commandments. Psalm 119:73 (NKJV)

Let my heart be blameless regarding Your statutes, That I may not be ashamed. Psalm 119:80 (NKJV)

The preface of the afflicted disciple's prayer contains a significant affirmation about the One who answers such prayers.

Preface means from *Webster's Encyclopedia Dictionary of the English Language*: a saying before hand; an introduction, to utter before hand, introductory remarks whether spoken or written. It is the opening statement at the beginning of a book explaining the reason for writing it. It is the initial and introductory part of the speech, leading up to, and preparing the way for the main portion which deals with some specific subject or arguments.

In this preface, he affirms that God's sovereign power had full sway over his being. The imagery of the LORD's "hands" speaks not only of power in general, but also, and especially in this context, of the creative dimensions of Divine omnipotence. Omnipotence means: state or quality of being able to do; having power and authority over all things; all-powerful almighty. God is omnipotent and Almighty God.

He indicates that God's hands "gave me my constitution," or as the NEB puts it: "made me what I am." Psalm 119:73 (NEB)

For You formed my inward parts; You covered me in my mother's womb. I will praise You, for I am fearfully and wonderfully made; Marvelous are Your works, And that my soul knows very well. My frame was not hidden from You, When I was made in secret, And skillfully wrought in the lowest parts of the earth. Your eyes saw my substance, being yet unformed. And in Your book they all were written, The days fashioned for me, When as yet there were none of them. Psalm 139:13-16 (NKJV)

You made me; You are my God, because of that you can get me through this. And as Sandra puts it: "If He cannot, then God can take me home to heaven to be with Him." The psalmist knew and understood that to which Jeremiah testifies:

"Before I formed you in the womb I knew you; Before you were born I sanctified you; I ordained you a prophet to the nations." Jeremiah 1:5 (NKJV)

Both the writer of Psalm 119 and Jeremiah knew that God knows us infinitely better than we know ourselves, since He has sovereignly overseen the framing of our personalities. It all begins with understanding God! In order to understand God we:

1. <u>Pray</u>: for spiritual growth towards maturity:

   Therefore, laying aside all malice, all deceit, hypocrisy, envy, and all evil speaking, as newborn babes, desire the pure milk of the word, that you may grow thereby, if indeed you have tasted that the LORD is gracious. 1 Peter 2:1-3 (NKJV)

2. <u>Pray</u>: for godly understanding, wisdom, knowledge and revelation.

   Repeated five times in the chapters of Psalm 119:

   Give me understanding, and I shall keep Your law; Indeed, I shall observe it with my whole heart. Psalm 119:34 (NKJV)

   Your hands have made me and fashioned me; Give me understanding, that I may learn Your commandments. Psalm 119:73 (NKJV)

   I am Your servant; Give me understanding, That I may know Your testimonies. Psalm 119:125 (NKJV)

   The righteousness of Your testimonies is everlasting; Give me understanding, and I shall live. Psalm 119:144 (NKJV)

   Let my cry come before You, O LORD; Give me understanding according to Your word. Psalm 119:169 (NKJV)

The psalmist cries out to God.

Blessed are You, O LORD! Teach me Your statutes. Psalm 119:12 (NKJV)

Open my eyes, that I may see Wondrous things from Your law Psalm 119:18 (NKJV)

I have declared my ways, and You answered me; Teach me Your statutes. Make me understand the way of Your precepts; So shall I meditate on Your wonderful works. Psalm 119:26-27 (NKJV)

Teach me, O LORD, the way of Your statutes, And I shall keep it to the end. Psalm 119:33 (NKJV)

Make me walk in the path of Your commandments, for I delight in it. Psalm 119:35 (NKJV)

The earth, O LORD, is full of Your mercy; Teach me Your statutes. Psalm 119:64 (NKJV)

Teach me good judgment and knowledge, For I believe Your commandments. Psalm 119:66 (NKJV)

Deal with Your servant according to Your mercy, And teach me Your statutes Psalm 119:124 (NKJV)

My eyes are awake through the night watches, That I may meditate on Your word. Psalm 119:148 (NKJV)

Salvation is far from the wicked, For they do not seek Your statutes. Psalm 119:155 (NKJV)

I rejoice at Your Word As one who finds great treasure. Psalm 119:162 (NKJV)

I hate and abhor lying, But I love Your law. Psalm 119:163 (NKJV)

Paul understood how God's grace helps us in our weakness.

I think you ought to know, dear brothers, about the hard time we went through in Asia. We were really crushed and overwhelmed, and feared we would never live through it. We felt we were doomed to die and saw how powerless we were to help ourselves; but that was good, for then we put everything into the hands of God, who alone could save us, for he can even raise the dead. And he did help us, and saved us from a terrible death; yes, and we expect him to do it again and again. 2 Corinthians 1:8-10 (TLB)

We are like clay jars in which this treasure is stored. The real power comes from God and not from us.

But we have this treasure in earthen vessels, that the excellence of the power may be of God and not of us. 2 Corinthians 4:7 (NKJV)

Because God made me, He can get me through any trial, temptation, suffering or struggle. It is this kind of understanding that drives the psalmist to the Source of answers. Not understanding as to why he is going through affliction, but answers as to how to undergo the affliction. God is the Master Mechanic, if you will; He has made us "the car" and He knows best how to fix us.

God is the Master Mechanic, and He through His Word wants to give us greater understanding that we may learn God's commandments. We can learn the easy way, by learning from other people's mistakes, as read in the Bible or we can learn the hard way, from making our own mistakes, it is our choice.

3. <u>Pray</u>: for discernment and sound judgment to apply God's Word to what is going on in our lives.

   Teach me good judgment and knowledge, For I believe Your commandments. Psalm 119:66 (NKJV)

A prayer for more discernment of God's special revelation resides in the heart of this verse.

4. <u>Pray</u>: for God to take you much further in His Word.
5. <u>Pray</u>: for God to help you hear, read, study, meditate, memorize scriptures and apply His Word to your life as He sees fit.
6. <u>Pray</u>: for conformity to the Word of God.

Conform means from *Webster's Encyclopedia Dictionary of the English Language*: to be in or bring into agreement; to comply.

Comply means: to yield or assent; to agree, to conform.

Note that the disciple is not merely focusing on external compliance, but especially on internal conformity—"Let my heart" (my very being of rational — easily moved; the nucleus of personality "be blameless" (in other words, sound or complete) "in Your statutes." He knew that outward conformity depended on inward conformity, so he prays that the very core of his being be perfectly compliant, meaning yielded and disposed to conformity with God's standards.

When troubles come, many times Christians pray, "Why is this happening to me?" or "Get me out of this!"

Versus and in contrast to:

"Give me understanding, that I may learn Thy commandments" and "May my heart be blameless in Thy statutes."

Do you detect the difference in these two attitudes in prayer? When we go through trial, may we pray for discernment of and conformity to the Word of God.

God wants to mature us in conformity with the standards of His lessons for life. He knows that mastering God's curriculum would provide the stability that we long for, especially in view of our trying circumstances.

In the following verses we see David turning to God and His Word, just like we should.

I thought about my ways, And turned my feet to Your testimonies. Psalm 119:59 (NKJV)

At midnight I will rise to give thanks to You, Because of Your righteous judgments. Psalm 119:62 (NKJV)

I rise before the dawning of the morning, And cry for help; I hope in Your word. Psalm 119:147 (NKJV)

Seven times a day I praise You, Because of Your righteous judgments. Psalm 119:164 (NKJV)

Evening and morning and at noon I will pray, and cry aloud, And He shall hear my voice. Psalm 55:17 (NKJV)

7. <u>Pray</u>: like David and give thanks to God.

Paul wrote:

Rejoice always, pray without ceasing, in everything give thanks; for this is the will of God in Christ Jesus for you. 1 Thessalonians 5:16-18 (NKJV)

The apostle Paul also wrote:

...giving thanks always for all things to God the Father in the name of our Lord Jesus Christ,... Ephesians 5:20 (NKJV)

God wants us to have and experience the fruit of the spirit called joy and peace. Then we will be able to thank God "in everything" "always " "in all things" without feelings of resentment, bitterness or regret. We are to be thankful for everything. It may not feel joyful while I am going through this suffering, but as Beth Moore says, "Joy has been appropriated to me so I choose joy."

In other words grant me practical perception for real life especially amidst its many pressures. This is spelled out clearly by the apostle James:

My brethren, count it all joy when you fall into various trials, knowing that the testing of your faith produces patience. But let patience have its perfect work, that you may be perfect and complete, lacking nothing. If any of you lacks wisdom, let him ask of God, who gives to all liberally and without reproach, and it will be given to him. But let him ask in faith, with no doubting, for he who doubts is like a wave of the sea driven and tossed by the wind. For let not that man suppose that he will receive anything from the Lord; he is a double-minded man, unstable in all his ways. James 1:2-8 (NKJV)

David turns his thoughts to other people. When faced with trials and sufferings we should pray for a positive testimony to other believers.

Those who fear You will be glad when they see me, Because I have hoped in Your word. Psalm 119:74 (NKJV)

8. Pray: to be a positive verbal and visual testimony to other believers. The psalmist's prayer is:

Let those who fear You turn to me, Those who know Your testimonies. Psalm 119:79 (NKJV)

People will be watching me while I go through suffering. The psalmist wishes all who fear God may see in him an example of the way in which trust in the Word of God is rewarded.

What is so important about this is, that, while he has every reason to be preoccupied with himself, he is thinking of others! When he prayed for himself, he prayed for spiritual maturity. When he prays for other believers, he prays for their "joy!" He wants them to be joyful and glad...because of his suffering? No. But, because while he is suffering, he waits for God's Word. They know full well of his plight, and he does not desire their pity, rather, he desires their encouragement. He wants his transparent life to reveal to those watching that he trusts truth in tribulation; that his hope and security are found in patiently waiting upon God.

The psalmist wants believers to "turn" to him for answers. And if the Hebrew text is not emended, the second part of the verse gives the purpose for their return—"that they may know Your testimonies." He wants to give them the reason for the hope that is within him. And that is that God's revelation is the sustaining power in his life.

Father, help us realize that the spotlight is brightest when trials and suffering flood our lives. Other Christians are watching to see how we handle hardships. If we are whining and saying "Why me?" or "Get me out of this!" then the testimony is not so positive. But, if we are resting on the promises of You, God, even when it appears all hope is gone then our witness is incredibly positive. "It brings gladness to the hearts of watching believers and it brings gladness to You, God, even when it appears all hope is gone then our witness is incredibly positive. It brings gladness to the hearts of watching believers and it brings gladness to You, God because it reaffirms to them and to You the basis of our hope! So when I am undergoing trial I pray that my restful patience in the promises of God will shine brightly to Your glory God. In Jesus Name, Amen.

9. <u>Pray</u>: to bear up under the weight of great suffering.

10. <u>Pray</u>: for godly perspective. The man of God acknowledges God's role in trials.

I know, O LORD, that Your judgments are right, And that in faithfulness You have afflicted me. Psalm 119:75 (NKJV)

He just comes out and says it. "You have afflicted me." And in so doing he recognizes two seemingly paradoxical truths about His LORD. God's judgments are righteous. His sovereign decisions and their executions and performance of it are righteous. Now, by itself, such an acknowledgement might seem like a polite theological concession. But he is not saying this in general, nor is he saying it to someone else. The psalmist says, "You have done it to me!" The reason this statement seems to be a paradox is, "if God's sovereign decisions and their execution are always perfectly right, then why am I experiencing affliction?" This is where most Christians stumble. If God is all-wise (He always does the right thing at the right time), and if God is sovereign (He is in total control of all that happens), and if He loves me, then why are bad things happening to me?

And we know that all things work together for good to those who love God, to those who are the called according to His purpose. Romans 8:28 (NKJV)

The psalmist is not asking "Why?" He knows that God is the Creator, and he knows that he is the creature. He knows that his thoughts are not God's thoughts and his ways are not God's way. So instead of trying to understand God, he rests in the fact that God's judgments are always righteous and that He is completely trustworthy—"in faithfulness You have afflicted me." God is faithful to the Covenant relationship; He will always chasten the disobedient or the negligent. But even if God does not answer your prayer in this lifetime "He helps us grow spiritually in our faith. God will bless the loyal servants. The psalmist knows that his punishment has been just and deserved, for God does not capriciously afflict His people.

11. <u>Pray</u>: to see this suffering from God's point of view, from His perspective.

> *Before I was afflicted I went astray, but now I keep Your word.* Psalm 119:67 (NKJV)

> *It is good for me that I have been afflicted, That I may learn Your statutes.* Psalm 119:71 (NKJV)

> *For He does not afflict willingly, Nor grieve the children of men.* Lamentations 3:33 (NKJV)

But David does not dwell on the punitive nature of inflicting punishment or the significance of his tribulations; rather, he focuses on the resultant benefit to himself. In other words:

> *And we know that all things work together for good to those who love God, to those who are the called according to His purpose.* Romans 8:28 (NKJV)

As Franz Delitzsch puts it, "He knows that God has humbled him, being faithful in His intentions toward him; for it is just in the school of affliction that one first learns rightly to estimate the worth of His Word, and comes to feel its power." Incidentally, God has other purposes for affliction besides correction. Affliction is sometimes used by God as a preventative measure, to keep us in the proper frame of mind, Paul said:

> *And lest I should be exalted above measure by the abundance of the revelations, a thorn in the flesh was given to me, a messenger of Satan to buffet me, lest I be exalted above measure. Concerning this thing I pleaded with the Lord three times that it might depart from me. And He said to me, "My grace is sufficient*

*for you, for My strength is made perfect in weakness."
Therefore most gladly I will rather boast in my infirmities,
that the power of Christ may rest upon me. Therefore I
take pleasure in infirmities, in reproaches, in needs, in
persecutions, in distresses, for Christ's sake. For when
I am weak, then I am strong.*
1 Corinthians 12:7-10 (NKJV)

Another purpose for affliction is sometimes for His glory.

> *Now as Jesus passed by, He saw a man who was
> blind from birth. And His disciples asked Him, saying
> "Rabbi, who sinned, this man or his parents, that
> he was born blind?" Jesus answered, "Neither this
> man nor his parents sinned, but that the works of
> God should be revealed in him.* John 9:1-3 (NKJV)
> (Rabbi means Teacher)

12. <u>Pray</u>: to recognize His glory.
13. <u>Pray</u>: acknowledge God's role, God's rule and God's reign.

> *You are good, and do good; Teach me Your stat-
> utes.* Psalm 119:68 (NKJV)

> *Forever, O LORD, Your word is settled in heaven.*
> Psalm 119:89 (NKJV)

> *Your faithfulness endures to all generations; You
> established the earth, and it abides.* Psalm 119:90
> (NKJV)

> *Your word is a lamp to my feet And a light to my
> path.* Psalm 119:105 (NKJV)

> *Make Your face shine upon Your servant, And teach
> me Your statutes.* Psalm 119:135 (NKJV)

Concerning Your testimonies, I have known of old that You have founded them forever. Psalm 119:152 (NKJV)

The entirety of Your word is truth, And every one of Your righteous judgments endures forever. Psalm 119:160 (NKJV)

Let my supplication come before You; Deliver me according to Your word. My lips shall utter praise, For You teach me Your statutes. My tongue shall speak of Your word, For all Your commandments are righteousness. Psalm 119:170-172(NKJV)

14. <u>Pray</u>: to acknowledge man's role in suffering.

May the arrogant be ashamed for they subvert me with a lie. Psalm 119:78 (NASB)

Arrogant—godless men—our enemies, God uses those people in our lives. God allowed but enemy is responsible. We see this in the life of Jesus.

"For truly against Your holy Servant Jesus, whom You anointed, both Herod and Pontius Pilate, with the Gentiles and the people of Israel, were gathered together to do whatever Your hand and Your purpose determined before to be done. Acts 4:27-28 (NKJV)

It was our fault too that Jesus suffered and died for our sins on the cross. Herod and Pontius Pilate were key participants, but we are all guilty of Christ's death on the cross. Silence killed Jesus— I learned that in the book, *Share Jesus without fear* by William Fay with Linda Evans Shepherd. No one spoke up for Jesus. Silence is still killing people. We will not open our mouths and tell people Jesus loves them and will forgive them for what they have done in their past if they only ask Him to forgive them. Jesus paid the sin penalty for you and me. I still sin. I still need God's forgiveness provided by Jesus' substitutionary death on the cross.

Let the proud be ashamed, For they treated me wrongfully with falsehood; But I will meditate on Your precepts. Psalm 119:78 (NKJV)

Although this man of God, the psalmist, recognized his LORD's sovereign sway over all things, especially his own affliction, he also understood that his enemies were none-the-less morally responsible and therefore deserving of retributive justice—the just punishment and penalty exacted for an injury.

Even though Herod and Pontius Pilate sentenced Jesus to death that does not excuse sinful actions of mankind. Men are responsible. It does not excuse our behavior, men are still responsible, and it does not get us off the hook. Jesus went to the cross willingly but Herod, Pontius Pilate, Annas and Caiaphas were still guilty and held accountable for putting Jesus there. But the fact that God sovereignly used them does not excuse our guilt. It does not excuse us just because it was God's plan. It does not excuse our sinful actions. They are responsible—we are responsible.

for all have sinned and fall short of the glory of God, Romans 3:23 (NKJV)

For whoever shall keep the whole law, and yet stumble in one point, he is guilty of all. For He who said, "Do not commit adultery," also said, "Do not murder." Now if you do not commit adultery, but you do murder, you have become a transgressor of the law. James 2:10-11 (NKJV)

Jesus said:

"You have heard that it was said to those of old, 'You shall not murder, and whoever murders will be in danger of the judgment.' But I say to you that whoever is angry with his brother without a cause shall be in danger of the judgment. And whoever says to his brother, 'Raca!' shall be in danger of the council. But whoever says, 'You fool!' shall be in danger of hell fire. Matthew 5:21-22 (NKJV)

We are all guilty of putting Jesus on the cross. It was our sins who put Him there. Each actor on the stage of human history is responsible for every scene of his role, and yet, the Divine Director, God, is standing backstage determining every detail of the production. Jews, Gentiles, King Herod and Pontius Pilate did an evil thing by crucifying an innocent man, Jesus. But, God used it to accomplish His predetermined plan. You do not have to feel like a victim. Do not think if you had been there it would have been any different. God was in control and Jesus chose to die on the cross to pay for our sins. We would not have spoken up either. But what about now? Can we change things; can we tell people about Jesus now? We do not have to be a part of the silent majority anymore.

People are still dying without knowing Christ today. They are still dying and going into an eternal hell because we still are not speaking up. We could not do anything about Jesus, He had to die, but we can tell others about the Jesus we love so they will not have to go to hell.

15. <u>Pray</u>: the most precious prayer there is; pray for forgiveness.

God will forgive us if we will only ask. God wipes out the trespass and sin held against us. Not guilty is written over our sin if you ask God for forgiveness and by believing in Jesus that He died for you.

In Genesis, the first book of the Bible, we read the story of Joseph, who was sold into slavery by his brothers. He ended up in Egypt. They told his Father, Jacob, that he was dead. But God worked it for good to save lives, even the lives of his family. But his brothers were none the less guilty. Look in Genesis chapters 37 and 39 through 50 for the whole account of the story. His brothers talked of killing Joseph but instead, because of jealousy, sold him into slavery. He was a slave to his master in Egypt. His master's wife harassed Joseph, and she falsely accused Joseph of rape for which he then was sentenced and thrown into prison for—years. Although Joseph helped others by interpreting their dreams they did not remember him until many years had passed. Pharaoh had a dream which needed to be interpreted, and Joseph was then remembered. He explained to Pharaoh the meaning of the dream, and Joseph was placed second in command to Pharaoh himself. This story in Genesis shows young men doing evil things, but all of it under God's control and for His purpose. Years later, in Egypt, Joseph's brothers had to stand before Joseph to ask for food for their family during a time of famine in Canaan and Egypt.

> *Joseph said to them: "Do not be afraid, for am I in the place of God? But as for you, you meant evil against me; but God meant it for good, in order to bring it about as it is this day, to save many people alive.* Genesis 50:19-20 (NKJV)

Joseph had a choice. He chose to forgive his brothers for what they did to him. Although this man of God recognized his LORD's sovereign sway over all things, especially including his own affliction, he also understood that his enemies were none-the-less morally responsible and therefore deserving of retributive justice, the just punishment and penalty exacted for an injury. Joseph chose to forgive his brothers.

I suppose that in the midst of any trial, we ought to ask "Why me?" For the spiritually immature, "Why me?" means "Why are You causing or allowing this to happen to me?" As if God is to blame. For the spiritually mature, "Why me?" means

"What are You trying to show me or teach me through this trial?" In the midst of any trial one should ask God, "What do You want me to do about this?" Or "What can I do that would honor You?" or "How can I be Your 'co-worker' in allowing this trial to conform me to the image of Christ?"

Here are some verses from Psalm 119 that speak to man's role:

I have done justice and righteousness; Do not leave me to my oppressors. Be surety for Your servant for good; Do not let the proud oppress me. Psalm 119:121-122 (NKJV)

It is time for You to act, O LORD, For they have regarded Your law as void. Psalm 119:126 (NKJV)

Redeem me from the oppression of man, That I may keep Your precepts. Psalm 119:134 (NKJV)

Many are my persecutors and my enemies, Yet I do not turn from Your testimonies. Psalm 119:157 (NKJV)

Princes persecute me without a cause, But my heart stands in awe of Your word. Psalm 119:161 (NKJV)

Seven times a day I praise You, Because of Your righteous judgments. Great peace have those who love Your law, And nothing causes them to stumble. LORD, I hope for Your salvation, And I do Your commandments. My soul keeps Your testimonies, And I love them exceedingly. I keep Your precepts and Your testimonies, For all my ways are before You.

Let my cry come before You, O LORD; Give me understanding according to Your word. Let my supplication come before You; Deliver me according to Your word.

My lips shall utter praise, For You teach me Your statutes. My tongue shall speak of Your word, For all Your commandments are righteousness.

Let Your hand become my help, For I have chosen Your precepts. I long for Your salvation, O LORD, And Your law is my delight. Let my soul live, and it shall praise You; And let Your judgments help me. Psalm 119:164-175 (NKJV)

God knows what we need already, but when we voice it to Him as a prayer and place it in His hands then and only then will He, (God), do something about it. God does nothing but in answer to prayer.

16. Pray: for help.

Let, I pray, Your merciful kindness be for my comfort, According to Your word to Your servant. Let Your tender mercies come to me, that I may live; For Your law is my delight. Psalm 119:76-77 (NKJV)

How do we survive times of suffering? We survive with God's help. That is what the psalmist prays for here.

Uphold me according to Your word, that I may live; And do not let me be ashamed of my hope. Hold me up, and I shall be safe, And I shall observe Your statutes continually. Psalm 119:116-117 (NKJV)

Direct my steps by Your word, And let no iniquity have dominion over me. Psalm 119:133 (NKJV)

I cry out with my whole heart; Hear me, O LORD! I will keep Your statutes. I cry out to You; Save me and I will keep Your testimonies. I rise before the dawning of the morning, And cry for help; I hope in Your word. Psalm 119:145-147 (NKJV)

Consider my affliction and deliver me, For I do not forget Your law. Psalm 119:153 (NKJV)

Let Your hand become my help, For I have chosen Your precepts. Psalm 119:173 (NKJV)

Let my soul live, and it shall praise You; And let Your judgments help me. I have gone astray like a lost sheep; Seek Your servant, For I do not forget Your commandments. Psalm 119:175-176 (NKJV)

You may not be able to voice your needs, but you can voice the shortest prayer there is: Help me, Jesus! Leave the "how" He helps You up to Him. Let go and put it into His hands to answer the best way He wants. Watch for His answer! God answers exceedingly abundantly above what we ask, think or can even imagine. God's ways are not our own ways nor His thoughts our thoughts.

Now to Him who is able to do exceedingly abundantly above all that we ask or think, according to the power that works in us, to Him be glory in the church by Christ Jesus to all generations, forever and ever. Amen. Ephesians 3:20-21 (NKJV)

"For My thoughts are not your thoughts, Nor are your ways My ways," says the LORD. "For as the heavens are higher than the earth, So are My ways higher than your ways, And My thoughts than your thoughts. Isaiah 55:8-9 (NKJV)

17. <u>Pray</u>: for God's comfort.

H. C. Leupoid summarizes the thrust of verse 76 in Psalm 119. "The one important fact that can always serve as a substantial comfort to those who suffer affliction is that God's steadfast love is the supreme comfort as God has promised that it will be." Notice here the Afflicter now becomes the Comforter! In this verse hope rises out of hurt, because amidst the tempestuous seas of this man's life his anchor gripped the great grace of God. Jeremiah the weeping prophet, whose life, from an earthly perspective was nothing but one huge failure, said this;

For the Lord will not cast off forever. Though He causes grief, Yet He will show compassion According to the multitude of His mercies. For He does not afflict willingly, Nor grieve the children of men. Lamentations 3:31-32 (NKJV)

God supplies according to the need. First Jeremiah prays for God's "hessed", unfailing, covenant keeping, and loyal love. In the Old Testament of the Bible "hessed" means faithful covenant keeping God. God, will never let us go. In the New Testament "charas" means grace. Jeremiah is saying, "Please let Your grace come." Why? "To comfort me." God's grace is greater than the need — grace upon grace, enough grace so we can give grace to someone else. You and I are forgiven when we ask, if we are Christians. Now it is our turn to forgive other people in our lives. Forgiveness is not a feeling. It is a mindset that leads to actions. It becomes loving actions toward someone who has wronged us. God forgave us; He expects us to forgive also. James reminds us in his epistle:

"But He gives more grace. Therefore He says: "God resists the proud, But gives grace to the humble." James 4:6 (NKJV)

Not only is grace greater than all our sins, but grace is greater than all our pain we are enduring, God's grace overwhelms the pain. Therein lies the comfort. (Bro. Randy said he cannot imagine any greater personal trial for him than losing his wife and children. That has not happened and he hopes it never will. However he has to believe that if and when that happens, the depth of his aching pain would be covered by God's infinite grace.)

18. <u>Pray</u>: for God's compassion.

Let Your tender mercies come to me, that I may live;
For Your law is my delight. Psalm 119:77 (NKJV)

The hurting child is pleading for his Heavenly Father's tender mercy. The Hebrew word for "compassion" refers to deep love (usually of a "superior" for an "inferior") rooted in some "natural" bond. The depth of this love is shown by the connection of this word "womb" Jeremiah uses it of a mother's love toward her nursing baby.

I am helpless as a baby and I am going under for the third time. It is breaking my heart that:

_____

_____

_____

_____

You fill in the blank. With what do you need help? You do not have to try to explain to God how he can help you. Simply voice your need to Him for His help and leave it up to Him how to answer. God can blow your mind with how He can come through for you when you ask Him in submission and obedience.

The verb, mercy, connotes a feeling which is most easily prompted by small babies or other helpless people. It incorporates the strong tie God has with His children.

Look upon me and be merciful to me, As Your custom is towards those who love Your name. Psalm 119:132 (NKJV)

19. <u>Pray</u>: for revival.

I learned from the book <u>Downpour</u> by James Macdonald, you cannot get re-vived (revived) and have revival in your soul until you have been "vived" and have Jesus in your heart, life, and have been born again. Then and only then can you ask for revival.

I have sworn and confirmed That I will keep Your righteous judgments. I am afflicted very much; Revive me, O LORD, according to Your word. Accept, I pray, the freewill offerings of my mouth, O LORD, And teach me Your judgments. Psalm 119:106-108 (NKJV)

Hear my voice according to Your loving kindness; O LORD, revive me according to Your justice. Psalm 119:149 (NKJV)

Plead my cause and redeem me; Revive me according to Your word. Psalm 119:154 (NKJV)

Great are Your tender mercies, O LORD; Revive me according to Your judgments. Psalm 119:156 (NKJV)

Consider how I love Your precepts; Revive me, O LORD, according to Your lovingkindness. Psalm 119:159 (NKJV)

(52)

Victory in the Valleys of Life

❧

*B*ro. Randy let me borrow his sermon notes from two funerals I attended. The messages spoke to my heart, and I hope they will speak to your heart as well. I have combined the notes from the two sermons into one. It explained to me and helped me understand my depression. And the Psalmist spoke to me how time and time again God had come along side me and nursed me back to health in all different ways.

Our Creator transcendent seeks to oversee six billion people on planet earth; but intimate so as to give constant vigil to me or you.

I learned about our galaxy from the *Crown Biblical Financial study-Life group manual*:

Astronomers estimate that there are more than 100 billion galaxies in the universe, each containing billions of stars. The distance from one end of a galaxy to the other is often measured in millions of light years. Though our sun is a relatively small star, it could contain more than one million earths, and it has temperatures of 20 million degrees at its center.

Bro. Randy spoke at the funeral:
Isaiah wrote,

> *Lift up your eyes on high, And see who has created these things, Who brings out their host by number; He calls them all by name, by the greatness of His might And the strength of His power; not one is missing.*
> Isaiah 40:26 (NKJV)

When you look up at the star-filled sky and realize that at least 250,000,000 X 250,000,000 stars, each larger than our sun, have been placed there by God's hand, it makes you feel pretty small and insignificant.

But when you realize that the Creator of this vast universe cares for you as an individual...you feel mighty special. In perhaps the most beloved of all passages in the Bible, a shepherd demonstrates that we are cared for individually.

Infinite, powerful, God of all creation, assumes toward His people the office and character of a Shepherd. We as sheep are weak, defenseless, and foolish, but God is our Provider, Preserver, Director, and He is everything to us!

Comfort and strength have come to more people in the hour of sorrow and death from the twenty-third Psalm than any other words ever penned. That is because it speaks to our deepest needs and our highest hopes.

The 23rd Psalm

> *The LORD is my shepherd; I shall not want.*

> *He makes me to lie down in green pastures; He leads me beside the still waters.*

> *He restores my soul; He leads me in the paths of righteousness For His name's sake.*

Yea, though I walk through the valley of the shadow of death, I will fear no evil; For You are with me; Your rod and Your staff, they comfort me.

You prepare a table before me in the presence of my enemies; You anoint my head with oil; My cup runs over.

Surely goodness and mercy shall follow me All the days of my life; And I will dwell in the house of the LORD Forever. Psalm 23:1-6 (NKJV)

David knew sheep. He knew that sheep were needy creatures. Left on their own, they were sure to fall and sure to fail. We need a Good Shepherd. David does not say, "The LORD is the shepherd of the world at large," but rather, "If He be a Shepherd to no one else, He is the Good Shepherd to me!" Perhaps the most precious word in verse one is the word "my." Is God a Good Shepherd to you? He is a prayer away.

Not "if," nor even "I hope so," but "is my Shepherd!" Do you belong to the LORD? This thought alone should stir our spirit, and lend enormous dignity to us as individuals of great importance to God. David was a shepherd. But here, he sees himself as a sheep. And, with a strong sense of pride, devotion, and admiration, he literally boasted aloud, "Look at who my shepherd is—my owner—my manager—my overseer. "It is the LORD Himself!"

Some of the wealthiest people, some of the most successful people, despite their outward show of success, despite their affluence and prestige, remain poor in spirit, shriveled in soul, unhealthy in life, under the ownership of the wrong master. Are you under the ownership of a cruel master? That can change today. Ask Jesus to save you and you can be under the ownership and tender mercy and care of the loving Shepherd, Jesus Christ. Then you will start understanding just how much the Great Shepherd, Jesus, cares for and comforts His helpless little sheep. Let's consider ways the Good Shepherd, Jesus, takes care of His sheep.

The Good Shepherd's provision suffices

Verses one and two:

> *The LORD is my shepherd; I shall not want. He makes me lie down in green pastures...(NKJV)*

There were pastures of fresh, tender, green grass. The original meaning was "a dwelling place, specifically an oasis; a verdant spot in the desert." The psalmist is communicating that the Good Shepherd provides for His sheep's physical needs—in this case food. Hungry sheep are ever on the move, always searching for green grass. A good shepherd knows where the grass is, and leads his sheep to that location. But while the provision of physical needs is alluded to, it is probably the provision of peace or contentment that is the primary thrust of the passage—"I shall not want" "He makes me lie down" which means to stretch oneself out, lie down, lie stretched out. God causes us to lie down.

David carries the thought of God's presence yielding peace to the flock, when he adds that He "leads me beside quiet waters." Lead is a pastoral word used of gentle leading; "still waters" are "quiet waters" which run deep. Not the torrent of a raging river, or the crashing waves of ocean tide, but the deep, peaceful streams of His abundance. Beside waters of refreshment He leads me and causes me to rest there.

When sheep are thirsty, they become restless and set out in search of water. If not led to the good water supplies of clean, pure water, they will often end up drinking from polluted potholes where they can pick up internal parasites.

When David composed this Psalm, he knew that the thirst of man could only be quenched in the deep, clear, still pools of God.

That is why Jesus said,

"If anyone thirsts, let him come to Me and drink." John 7:37 (NKJV)

Often the deep waters of God are found in places of great inaccessibility. Phillip Kellar tells of standing under the blazing equatorial sun of Africa and watching the native herds being led to their owner's water wells. Some of these were enormous, hand hewn caverns out of the sandstone formations along the rivers. They were like great rooms chiseled out of the rocks with ramps running down to the water trough at the bottom. The herds and flocks were led down into these deep cisterns where cool, clear, clean water awaited them.

In the Christian's life, many of the places we may be led into will appear to us as dark, deep, dangerous, and somewhat disagreeable. But it simply must be remembered that He is there with us. God is very much at work in the situation if you have prayed and asked Him. It is His energy, effort and strength expended on our behalf that causes even this deep, dark place to produce a benefit for us.

Sheep are timid and sheep are nervous. Even the slightest suspicion of a predator leaves them anxious. Left alone they would probably spend a lot of their time darting about aimlessly, not knowing where they are going or why they are going, but just going! The sheep of God's pasture can rest easy because they are aware of the constant, abiding presence of the Good Shepherd.

Sheep can be driven to absolute distraction by flies and ticks. Instead of lying down to rest, they are up on their feet, stomping their feet and shaking their heads. We as Christians, because we do not understand all of God's plans, sometimes act like that towards God. We want things to go our way but sometimes that is not the best way and we become distracted by the annoying things that happen in our lives. Our Shepherd is faithful. In the ancient Middle East, where there were no barbed wire fences, shepherds would construct sheep folds out of rocks. These sheep folds had only one entrance. At the end of a day of grazing, the shepherd called the sheep into the sheep fold. He would stand at this opening, applying oil to wounds and sores so that flies and parasites would not bother the sheep.

The Good Shepherd's presence sustains—He sustains by restoring us.

Verse three:

"He restores my soul; He leads me in the path of righteousness for His name sake. (NKJV)

An old English Shepherd's term for a sheep that has turned over on its back and cannot get up again by itself is, "cast, or cast down." A heavy long-fleeced sheep will sometimes lie down on an incline or in some little hollow in the ground. It may roll on its side slightly to stretch out or relax and end up on its back. Suddenly, the center of gravity in the body shifts so that it turns on its back far enough that the feet no longer touch the ground. It may feel a sense of panic and start to paw frantically. Frequently, this only makes matters worse. It rolls over even further. Now it is impossible to get back on its feet. Gases build up in the rumen and circulation is cut off to the extremities. If the predators do not kill it, the elements will. When the shepherd finds this one out of 99, who has strayed and become "cast down," he rolls it on its side, to relieve the pressure of the gases in the rumen, and then rubs its legs until circulation is restored. The shepherd then restores it to an upright position, and it joins the 99 other sheep.

Many people have the idea that when a child of God falls, when he is frustrated and helpless, God becomes disgusted, fed-up, and even angry. David says, "He restores my soul." When the soul grows sorrowful, He revives it. When it is weak, He strengthens it. When it is sinful, He forgives and sanctifies it. When we are cast down, God sets us on our feet again. God does it. The presence of the shepherd sustains the sheep. When we read the life story of Jesus, we see Him again and again, picking up "cast sheep."

David knew what it was to be cast down and dejected. He had tasted defeat in his life and felt frustration at having fallen into temptation. David was acquainted with the bitterness of feeling hopeless and without strength in himself.

The Good Shepherd sustains us by guiding us, He sustains us by restoring us. And He sustains us through His guidance.

Left to our own devices, we would go astray. The Good Shepherd guides us. He is not an "absentee owner"—checking on the flock only occasionally; He travels the path with us.

The Good Shepherd sustains by protecting us.
Verse four:

> *"Yea, though I walk through the valley of the shadow of death, I will fear no evil."* (NKJV)

The "valley of the shadow of death" is any time of dread and darkness. The psalmist does not say, "if I go through," but "though I walk through." He knows there will be tough times in his life. And he does not say, "Though I stay in the valley of the shadow of death." He says, "Though I walk <u>through</u> the valley of the shadow of death." And the psalmist does not say, "The valley of death;" he says, "The valley of the <u>shadow</u> of death." But most noteworthy is how he makes it: "For You art with me; Your rod and Your staff, they comfort me." The presence of the Good Shepherd gets the sheep through tough times.

David does not linger long in green pastures or beside the still waters. He moves quickly to the dark valleys of life.

Here is the picture—the flock, under the watchful eye of the shepherd, moves miles from their summer pastures up into the high rangelands. All the dangers of rampaging rivers in flood stage, avalanches, rock-slides, predators, and spring storms await the moving flock.

We do not live long until we realize that life has many dark valleys. Sickness is a valley. Loneliness is a valley. Depression is a valley. Failure is a valley. Divorce is a valley. And death is a valley.

What gives the sheep assurance in the dreads of life? The presence of the Shepherd—

verse four continues,

"for Thou art with me."(KJV)

Not that He is waiting on the other side of the valley, urging me forward, while I am being singed by the fires of trial, but that He is my personal fire-ring, my asbestos suit now. David knows that the sheep are better off in the valley with the Good Shepherd, than-on-the mountain top alone!

Because of the Shepherd's presence and because of the Shepherd's power David does not view it as "the valley of death," but rather, as "the valley of the <u>shadow</u> of death."

Shadows have no substance. The substance of death has been removed, and only the shadow remains. Someone has said that when there is a shadow, there must be light some-where, and so there is. A shadow is ominous and causes fear, but the reason for fear lacks substance. A shadow cannot stop a man's pathway, even for a moment. The shadow of a dog cannot bite; the shadow of a sword cannot kill; the shadow of death cannot destroy. Therefore, let us not fear! Although evil is real, it is not victorious over the sheep in God's flock. Even the last enemy—death—has been conquered. And because of the victory that God's sheep have over the last and greatest enemy, they should fear no lesser enemy. I will look upon the last enemy as a conquered foe.

Donald Grey Barnhouse was a prince among American Presbyterian clergymen in the first half of the twentieth cen-tury. His first wife died from cancer while still in her thirties, leaving him with three children under the age of twelve. He had such victory that he decided to preach his wife's funeral service himself. The day of the funeral, Barnhouse and his children were driving to the funeral service when they were overtaken by a large truck, which, as it passed by, cast a large shadow over the car. Turning to his oldest daughter, who was staring sadly out the window of the car, Barnhouse asked, "Tell me, sweetheart, would you rather be run over by a truck or by its shadow? Looking curiously at her father, she replied, "By the shadow, I guess. It cannot hurt you." Speaking to all of his children, he said, "Your mother has not been overridden by death, but by the shadow of death. That is nothing to fear."

The Good Shepherd's preparation sustains.

Verses five and six:

> *You prepare a table before me in the presence of my enemies; You anoint my head with oil; My cup runs over, Surely goodness and mercy shall follow me All the days of my life;* (NKJV)

With these verses, there is an obvious change in imagery. We have moved from the pasture to a palace. And God, who was portrayed as the Good Shepherd, is now pictured as the Gracious Host.

In David's day, it was customary for Bedouin sheikhs to invite any wanderer passing his tent to be his guest for up to three days. At the end of this time the sheikh accompanies the traveler to the border of his territory and is no longer responsible for his guest.

David is taking the desert custom of hospitality extended towards a weary and endangered traveler to a new level of understanding. David elevates this custom to a spiritual level—"in the valley of the shadow of death," not a Bedouin, but God Himself prepares a table before me, anoints my head with oil, and fills my cup to overflowing. The Good Shepherd is also the Gracious Host. But there is a difference between the hospitality of the Bedouin sheikh and God. The Bedouin sheikh hosts for three days; God hosts forever! The promise extends into eternity!

Verse six:

I will dwell in the house of the LORD forever. (NKJV)

The word dwell means "to settle down and be at home with." When we come to the end of the dark valley, there is peace and plenty in His palace forever. Our assurance in the face of death is that beyond the valley of shadows is the Father's house. We have His word on that. This is not wishful thinking; it is a divine guarantee. His promise is certain. The Hebrew word "surely" is a word for certainty. Our assurance, in the face of death, is that beyond the valley of the shadows is the Father's house. We have His word on it.

David was an old man when he wrote this psalm. He has seen tragedy, disappointment, heartache, and death. But he had found in the LORD the grace and strength he needed to keep going. We can also. His provision suffices, His presence sustains; His preparation secures.

Think of it:

Beneath me: green pastures; Beside me: still waters; Before me: goodness and mercy; And beyond me: the Father's house. And throughout the entire journey, the Shepherd with me.

Amazing Grace! How sweet the sound
Words by John Newton

Amazing grace! How sweet the sound, that saved a wretch like me! I once was lost, but now am found, was blind, but now I see. Twas grace that taught my heart to fear, And grace my fears relieved; How precious did that grace appear The hour I first believed! Thro' many dangers, toils and snares, I have already come; Tis grace hath brought me safe thus far, And grace will lead me home. The LORD has promised good to me, His word my hope secures; He will my shield and portion be As long as life endures. When we've been there ten thousand years, Bright shining as the sun, We've no less days to sing God's praise Than when we first begun. Amen.

(53)

TEST-I-MONY

ॐ

$\mathcal{N}$otice the "I" in the middle of testimony. I can share my testimony of what God has done in my life with other people and you can too. Will you? It is so important to share your testimony with others so lost people can come to know the Jesus you know.

Pray for a positive visual and verbal testimony. It is important to live godly lives so even when we are silent, others will see us live out day by day our faith in Christ.

I have asked God for a positive testimony in writing, I know I need His help.

In chapter 39 of <u>Purpose Driven Life</u>, Rick Warren, who wrote the book explains the need for balance in the Christian life. He also encourages Christians to write down our progress in a journal which is the best way to reinforce progress in fulfilling God's purposes. This is not a diary of events, but a record of the life lessons you do not want to forget. The Bible says:

It is crucial that we keep a firm grip on what we've heard so that we do not drift off. Hebrews 2:1 (The Message Bible)

Rick Warren writes: We remember what we record. Writing helps clarify what God is doing in our lives. Dawson Trotman used to say, "Thoughts disentangle themselves when they pass through your fingertips." The Bible has several examples of God telling people to keep a spiritual journal. It says:

Now Moses wrote down the starting points of their journeys at the command of the LORD... Numbers 33:2 (NKJV)

Moses recorded the stages in their journey, at the LORD's command. Aren't you glad Moses obeyed God's command to record Israel's spiritual journey? If he had been lazy, we would be robbed of the powerful life lessons of the Exodus. While it is unlikely that your spiritual journal will be as widely read as Moses' was, yours is still important. Your life is a journey, and a journey deserves a journal. I hope you will write about the stages of your spiritual journey in living a purpose driven life. Do not just write down the pleasant things. As David did, record your doubts, fears, and struggles with God. Our greatest lessons come out of pain, and the Bible says:

You number my wanderings; Put my tears into Your bottle: Are they not in Your book? Psalm 56:8 (NKJV)

Whenever problems occur, remember that God uses them to fulfill all five purposes in your life: Problems force you to focus on God, draw you closer to others in fellowship, build Christ like character, provide you with a ministry, and give you a testimony. Every problem is purpose-driven. In the middle of a painful experience, the psalmist wrote,

This will be written for the generation to come, That a people yet to be created may praise the LORD. Psalm 102:18 (NKJV)

You owe it to future generations to preserve the testimony of how God helped you fulfill His purposes on earth. It is a witness that will continue to speak long after You are in heaven. If you want to keep growing, the best way to learn more is to pass on to others what you have already learned.

The one who blesses others is abundantly blessed; those who help others are helped. Proverbs 11:25 (The Message Bible)

Those who pass along insights get more from God. It is all for God's Glory! The reason we pass on what we learn is for the glory of God and the growth of his kingdom. The night before He was crucified, Jesus reported to His Father,

"I have brought you glory on earth by completing the work you gave me to do. John 17:4 (NIV)

When Jesus prayed these words, He had not yet died for our sins, so what "work" had He completed? In this instance He was referring to something other than the atonement. The answer lies in what He said in the next twenty-three verses of His prayer.

Jesus is speaking:

"But now I go away to Him who sent Me, and none of you asks Me, 'Where are You going?' But because I have said these things to you, sorrow has filled your heart. Nevertheless I tell you the truth. It is to your advantage that I go away; for if I do not go away, the Helper will not come to you; but if I depart, I will send Him to you. And when He has come, He will convict the world of sin, and of righteousness, and of judgment: of sin, because they do not believe in Me, of righteousness, because I go to My Father and you see Me no

more; of judgment, because the ruler of this world is judged.

"I still have many things to say to you, but you cannot bear them now. However, when He, the Spirit of truth, has come, He will guide you into all truth; for He will not speak on His own authority, but whatever He hears He will speak; and He will tell you things to come. He will glorify Me, for He will take of what is Mine and declare it to you. All things that the Father has are Mine. Therefore I said that He will take of Mine and declare it to you.

"A little while, and you will not see Me; and again a little while, and you will see Me, because I go to the Father."

Then some of His disciples said among themselves, "What is this that He says to us, 'A little while, and you will not see Me; and again a little while, and you will see Me"; and. 'because I go to the Father'?" They said therefore, "What is this that He says, 'A little while'? We do not know what He is saying."

Now Jesus knew that they desired to ask Him, and He said to them, "Are you inquiring among yourselves about what I said, 'A little while, and you will not see Me; and again a little while and you will see Me'? Most assuredly, I say to you that you will weep and lament, but the world will rejoice; and you will be sorrowful, but your sorrow will be turned into joy. A woman, when she is in labor, has sorrow because her hour has come; but as soon as she has given birth to the child, she no longer remembers the anguish, for joy that a human being has been born into the world. Therefore you now have sorrow; but I will see you again and your heart will rejoice, and your joy no one will take from you.

And in that day you will ask Me nothing. Most assuredly, I say to you, whatever you ask the Father in My name He will give you. Until now you have asked nothing in My name. Ask, and you will receive, that your joy may be full.

"These things I have spoken to you in figurative language; but the time is coming when I will no longer speak to you in figurative language, but I will tell you plainly about the Father. In that day you will ask in My name, and I do not say to you that I shall pray the Father for you, for the Father Himself loves you, because you have loved Me, and have believed that I came forth from God. I came forth from the Father and have come into the world. Again I leave the world and go to the Father." John 16:5-28 (NKJV)

Jesus told His Father what He had been doing for the last three years: preparing His disciples to live for God's purposes. He helped them to know and love God (worship), taught them to love each other (fellowship), gave them the Word so they could grow to maturity (discipleship), showed them how to serve (ministry), and sent them out to tell others (mission). Jesus modeled a purpose-driven life, and He taught others how to live it, too. That was the "work" that brought glory to God. Today God calls each of us to the same work. Not only does He want us to live out His purposes, He also wants us to help others do the same. God wants us to introduce people to Christ, bring them into His fellowship, and help them grow to maturity and discover their place of service, and then send them out to reach others too. This is what purpose-driven living is all about. Regardless of your age, the rest of your life can be the best of your life, and you can start living on purpose today.

Why I Wrote

I found all the verses in the Bible to be my example for this prayer of being a positive testimony in writing. If people had not written the scripture, we would not have the Bible today. It may not be a whole book like this; it may be just short notes in a journal. Even journaling my prayers over the years prepared me to write now.

This book has mainly been written to lost people; people who may not even own a Bible. Now I am addressing the saved? The psalmist cried out to God for revival. Do you want revival? Then it has to start with one—you. You have to ask it for yourself. Revival may not come because it is on the calendar of your church—it can come that way. But it continues as we cry out to God to continue to revive us. Are you tired? The first thing God may have you do is rest and eat; rest and eat; rest and eat just like Bro. Randy suggested I do two years ago during spring break. Then maybe you can find some time to play like Dr. Snowden suggested. But it involves worship also. Read God's word, pray and go to church. Then as you get more joy back in your life and are stronger, invest your life in loving some other people God has or will place in your life.

Bro Randy and Pam suggested that I read *The Five Love Languages for Singles* by Gary Chapman. The book also comes in a couple's version and a version for teenagers. God is not here so we can physically love Him. We are to love the people in our lives to practice and learn how to love until we meet God face to face. The book says different people receive love in one or more of five different ways: Words of Affection; Gifts; Acts of service; Quality time and Physical touch. Loving in the way a person receives it has dramatically changed my relationship with my Momma and Daddy. Also I recommend you see the movie *Fireproof*. It goes along with the *Love Dare* book but it also is in complement with the *Five Love Languages* book. So until you see God face to face and can love Him physically—love other people. The books I suggested for you to read can help you with how to love.

Jesus tells us:

> *And the King will answer and say to them, 'Assuredly, I say to you, inasmuch as you did it to one of the least of these My brethren, you did it to Me.'* Matthew 25:40 (NKJV)

(55)

How to Face Persecution

O ctober 24, 2009 Bro. Randy's morning sermon based on Daniel 6: 1-28. It taught me I will be persecuted and what my response should be.

Paul says,

"Indeed, all who desire to live godly in Christ Jesus will be persecuted."

"in labors more abundant, in stripes above measure, in prisons more frequently, in deaths often. From the Jews five times I received forty stripes minus one., Three times I was beaten with rods, once I was stoned...in perils of robbers, in perils of my own countrymen, in perils of the Gentiles, in perils in the city...in the wilderness...on the sea...among false brethren," (2 Corinthians 11:23-26 (NKJV)

The writer of Hebrews (possibly Paul) shares with us, in the 11th chapter, the Christians martyr "Hall of Fame."

Others were tortured, not accepting deliverance, that they might obtain a better resurrection. Still others had trial of mocking and scourging, yes, and of chains and imprisonment. They were stoned, they were sawn in two, were tempted, were slain with the sword. They wandered about in sheepskins and goatskins, being destitute, afflicted, tormented—of whom the world was not worthy. They wandered in deserts and mountains, in dens and caves of the earth. Hebrews 11:36-38 (NKJV)

Isaiah believed God, and he was sawn in half; Paul believed God and he was decapitated; Peter believed God and was crucified upside down. Believing God does not necessarily guarantee you that you will not be sliced and diced, or, in the case of Daniel, to be put in the lion's den.

Before Bro. Randy and Pam had children, they kind of adopted a young man who was serving as a summer-time missionary to the visitors at a local park. Every day the young man would visit the campers staying there. Most of his attempts to share the gospel were met with apathy, some with anger and rebuffing. Bro. Randy asked him one day how he coped with the rejection. He said this: "It is not being persecuted that bothers me; what would bother me is if I were not being persecuted."

"All who desire to live godly in Christ Jesus will be persecuted."

It is tough to live godly in an ungodly world. But if we cannot even do so in the face of teasing, rejection, and ostracizing, how could we ever expect to in the face of scourging, stoning and the lions den? The story of Daniel and the lions den is perhaps the most famous story in the Bible—maybe even in the history of mankind regarding persecution.

How to act until the persecution comes:

It pleased Darius to set over the kingdom one hundred and twenty satraps, to be over the whole kingdom; and over these, three governors, of whom Daniel was one, that the satraps might give account to them, so that the king would suffer no loss. Then this Daniel distinguished himself above the governors and satraps, because an excellent spirit was in him; and the king gave thought to setting him over the whole realm. Daniel 6:1-3 (NKJV)

The lions are often the "stars of the show." So in our haste to get to the den, we bypass the palace. We should not, because therein we get a clue as to the kind of man Daniel was. "the king planned to appoint him over the entire kingdom," (v. 3b) The King James Version of the Bible puts it this way: "He was preferred." That word "preferred" in the original Aramaic, has in it a meaning, "He outshone them all." There was a light in Daniel not found in the other counselors and cabinet members. Why was he preferred? Because "he possessed an extraordinary spirit, (v.3). He was no doubt recognized as outstanding by the king, but apparently had that reputation throughout the kingdom as a whole. At least the Queen Mother, probably his Grandmother, described him to Belshazzar that way, (There is no word for grandmother or grandfather in the language of the Bible so the Queen Mother could have been his Grandmother)

There is a man in your kingdom in whom is the Spirit of the Holy God. And in the days of your father, light and understanding and wisdom, like the wisdom of the gods, were found in him; and King Nebuchadnezzar your father—your father the king—made him chief of the magicians, astrologers, Chaldeans, and soothsayers. Inasmuch as an excellent spirit, knowledge, understanding, interpreting dreams, solving riddles,

and explaining enigmas were found in this Daniel,
Daniel 5:11-12a (NKJV)

Although Daniel is now approaching ninety years of age, there's "an extraordinary spirit about him." W. A. Criswell says, "There is a youthfulness about him. There is a hopefulness about him. There is a spirit of optimism about him, and it is contagious. This Daniel, almost ninety years of age, is still in soul and in spirit, living the life of a young man." Daniel was a man with an extraordinary spirit.

In chapter 1 of the book of Daniel, as a teenager, he refused the king's food for consciences sake. In chapter 2, where Nebuchadnezzar threatens to kill all the wise men of the kingdom, of whom Daniel is one, he remains composed in the crisis, he's confident in prayer, he's courageous before men, and he's contrite in spirit. In chapter 4, he tells Nebuchadnezzar the truth, although the news is not good. Furthermore, he most likely runs the kingdom while Nebuchadnezzar's eating grass on his knees for seven years. And, in chapter 5, he refuses Belshazzar's gifts, and delivers the message of judgment unflinchingly. Daniel is never found complaining. He is a captive. He is a slave. He was removed from his home as a teenager, and in all likelihood, castrated, so as to serve as a eunuch in the king's palace. Daniel had an extraordinary spirit.

Apparently most, if not all the government officials, were jealous of Daniel, so they scrutinized his job and personal life for flaws. "Jealousy is the tribute that mediocrity pays to genius." In every judgment he made, every deed he did, every manuscript he signed, every order he gave as he governed the kingdom—in these they looked for wrongdoing. They found no fault in him. He was above bribery. Had Daniel been open to a bribe, had he one eye open as he held the scales of justice, had he closed his mouth when he should be speaking out, had there been any fault in him, they would have seized upon it immediately. But he was impeccable. He was incorruptible. He was a man of integrity, honesty, nobility, and purity. No neglect—there was not anything that he should have done, that he did not. No corruption—there was not anything that he should not have done, that he did. No act of commission, nor any act of omission.

So the governors and satraps sought to find some charge against Daniel concerning the kingdom; but they could find no charge or fault, because he was faithful; nor was there any error or fault found in him.
Daniel 6:4 (NKJV)

Alexander McLaren said, "It is remarkable that a character of such beauty and consecration as Daniel's should be rooted and grow out of the court where Daniel was. For this court was half shambles and half pig sty. It was filled with luxury and sensuality and lust and self-seeking and idolatry and ruthless cruelty. And the like was the environment of this man. And in the middle of this there grew up that fair flower of character, pure and stainless by the acknowledging of his enemies." Daniel, in that environment shone brightly to the testimony of the grace of God. And when his enemies took their searchlights, looking for something wrong in him, they did not succeed. When you read through the Old Testament, you will find only three men of whom nothing negative is said: One is Joseph, another is Jonathan, the pure, magnanimous, friend of David. And the third is Daniel. When faced with the threat of persecution, Daniel shows us how to live.

There was only one way to get him. He worshipped Jehovah. They did not.

Then these men said, "We shall not find any charge against this Daniel unless we find it against him concerning the law of his God."

So these governors and satraps thronged before the king, and said thus to him: "King Darius live forever! All the governors of the kingdom, the administrators and satraps, the counselors and advisors, have consulted together to establish a royal statute and to make a firm decree, that whoever petitions any god or man for thirty days, except you, O king, shall be cast into the den of lions. Now, O king, establish the decree and sign the writing, so that it cannot be changed, according to the laws of the Medes and Persians, which does not alter." Therefore King Darius signed the written decree. Daniel 6:5-9 (NKJV)

How to react after the persecution arrives:

Now when Daniel knew that the writing was signed, he went home. And in his upper room, with his windows open toward Jerusalem, he knelt down on his knees three times that day, and prayed and gave thanks before his God, as was his custom since early days.

Then these men assembled and found Daniel praying and making supplication before his God. And they went before the king, and spoke concerning the king's decree: "Have you not signed a decree that every man who petitions any god or man within thirty days, except you, O king, shall be cast into the den of lions?"

The king answered and said, "The thing is true, according to the law of the Medes and Persians, which does not alter."

So they answered and said before the king, "That Daniel, who is one of the captives from Judah, does not show due regard for you, O king, or for the decree that you have signed, but makes his petition three times a day." Daniel 6:10-13 (NKJV)

Daniel did not do anything when he found out that the decree had been written, except what he was accustomed to doing. When the pressure was on, he did not change! The greatest characteristics of godliness in the life of a person—that they can move through the vicissitudes of life, untouched by the circumstances that life throws at them...unaffected. When Daniel knew of the decree, and that it was signed, he remained just the same—unperturbed, without anxiety or foreboding, just kneeling in the presence of his great God.

When they sin against You (for there is no one who does not sin), and You become angry with them and deliver them to the enemy, and they take them captive to the land of the enemy, far or near; yet when they come to themselves in the land where they were carried captive, and repent, and make supplication to You in the land of those who took them captive, saying, "We have sinned and done wrong, we have committed wickedness'; and when they return to You with all their heart and with all their soul in the land of their enemies who led them away captive, and pray to You toward their land which You gave to their fathers, the city which You have chosen and the temple which I have built of Your name: then hear in heaven Your dwelling place their prayer and their supplication, and maintain their cause, and forgive Your people who have sinned against You, and all their transgressions which they have transgressed against You; and grant them compassion before those who took them captive, that then I may have compassion on them (for they are Your people and Your inheritance, whom You brought out of Egypt, out of the iron furnace), that Your eyes may be open to the supplication of Your servant and the supplication of Your people Israel, to listen to them whenever they call to You. 1 Kings 8:46-52 (NKJV)

"Toward their land"—Saying by their posture in prayer that God could be believed that He would return them to their land.

We are reactors. When the circumstances heat up we react with uncertainty and anxiety. Daniel teaches us that no matter what happens just go forward. Daniel would rather be thrown to the lions, because of the fear of God, than to acquiesce to save his own neck. He has not changed one bit since he was a teenager.

When they burned Polycarp at the stake in Smyrna in A.D. 155, he had been a Christian for eighty-six years. Much martyrdom had taken place before he was finally martyred. At the martyrdom of Germanius, the howling mob cried, "Away with the atheists." (They thought that the Christians were the atheists) "Let Polycarp be sought out." Polycarp was urged by his friends to seek refuge. He did for a time, and while doing so, he prayed. While praying, he had a vision that the pillow beneath his head was on fire. He interpreted this as the method of his death. Although he could have escaped, he did not so choose. When his accusers came for him, they said, "What harm is there in saying, 'Lord Caesar'?" He would not do it. He went to the stadium, and one of the judges pleaded, "Polycarp, have respect for your age. Repent and say, 'Away with the atheists.'" Polycarp looked across the stadium, and pointing at his accusers, he said, "Away with the atheist." The proconsul said, "Swear and I will set thee at liberty; reproach Christ." Before they lit the fire they called on Polycarp to deny the Lord and save his life. In quiet assurance and with steady voice he said: "Eight and six years have I served Him, and He hath done me no harm. How then could I blaspheme my King and my Savior?" They said, "We'll just burn you." And he said, "The fire you have for me will burn but for one hour; the fire for you will burn forever!" The account of his martyrdom reports that the fire that they made for him would not burn him to death. So finally, one of the executioners stuck a dagger in him to kill him.

The key to Daniel's life is found in Daniel 1:21. "And Daniel continued...He was consistent in spirit ("excellent in spirit") and he had a good attitude, there was no grumbling, no complaining and no wrangling. He was consistent in performance ("faithful man") and dependable. He did what he said he would do, he was credible and believable. Daniel was consistent in purity—highest government officials searched for flaws and could not find any: "no fault" "no corruption" "no error" "no neglect". Daniel was consistent in prayer (Read Daniel chapters 2, 4, and 9)

Daniel prayed as he always did:

Faith: toward Jerusalem
Humility: on his knees
Petition: asking petitions
Praise: giving thanks

What to expect during persecution:

There is a probability of the lion's den.

The nature of the Christian faith marks all of us for the "lions." We are out of step with the world around us. When Shadrach, Meshach, and Abed-Nego stood as everyone else bowed to the image which Nebuchadnezzar had erected they were marked for the fiery furnace. (see chapter 3 of Daniel) Notice God delivered the three young men through the fiery furnace. Now Daniel is kneeling while all others are standing. Notice God delivers Daniel through the lion's den. There was no attempt on the part of God to withhold them from the pressure of certain death. Every Christian will face the lions. Satan is like a roaring lion prowling around seeking whom he may devour.

So the king gave the command, and they brought Daniel and cast him into the den of lions. But the king spoke, saying to Daniel, "Your God, whom you serve continually, He will deliver you," Then a stone was brought and laid on the mouth of the den, and the king sealed it with his own signet ring and with the signets of his lords, that the purpose concerning Daniel might not be changed.

Now the king went to his palace and spent the night fasting; and no musicians were brought before him. Also his sleep went from him. Then the king arose very early in the morning and went in haste to the den of lions. And when he came to the den, he cried out with a lamenting voice to Daniel. The king spoke, saying to Daniel, "Daniel, servant of the living God has your God, whom you serve continually, been able to deliver you from the lions?"

Then Daniel said to the king, "O king, live forever! My God sent His angel and shut the lions mouths, so that they have not hurt me, because I was found innocent before Him; and also, O king, I have done no wrong before you."

Now the king was exceedingly glad for him, and commanded that they should take Daniel up out of the den. So Daniel was taken up out of the den, and no injury whatever was found on him, because he believed in his God. Daniel 6:16-23 (NKJV)

There is a deliverance from evil.

Some say that he snuck in the lion's den, or that he hid in the corner, or some other "logical" explanation.

And the king gave the command, and they brought those men who accused Daniel, and they cast them into the den of lions—them, their children, and their wives; and the lions overpowered them, and broke all their bones in pieces before they ever came to the bottom of the den. Daniel 6:24 (NKJV)

They (122 princes and two others and their families; about 300 to 400 people) were devoured before they hit the floor! There were lots of lions. All those who had persecuted Daniel were themselves persecuted. Like Haman who was hanged on his own gallows. And in Acts 12: Herod stretched his hand forth to get the church, and God stretched His hand forth and got Herod- Herod was eaten of worms and died.

He made a pit and dug it out, And has fallen into the ditch which he made. Psalm 7:15 (NKJV)

The child of God will ultimately and completely be delivered from evil. Remember what Jesus taught us to pray? "but deliver us from evil (the evil one)." Well it will be accomplished! "All's well that ends well." Well it all ends well for the child of God! Grace will always cover suffering.

No temptation has overtaken you except such as is common to man; but God is faithful, who will not allow you to be tempted beyond what you are able, but with the temptation will also make the way of escape, that you may be able to bear it. 1 Corinthians 10:13 (NKJV)

If you die, you go home to heaven sooner!

You who love the LORD, hate evil! He preserves the souls of His saints; He delivers them out of the hand of the wicked. Psalm 97:10 (NKJV)

"A man of God in the will of God is immortal until his work on earth is done." As long as I am a man of God doing the will of God, nothing on earth can touch me until God's done with me.

Daniel was not kept from the lion's den but in it.

The angel of the LORD encamps all around those who fear Him, And delivers them. Psalm 34:7 (NKJV)

Was "his angel" the same One who stood with Shadrach, Meshach, and Abed-Nego in the fiery furnace? A teacher asked a group of girls why Daniel was not afraid in the lion's den, and one little girl answered, "Because one of the lions was the Lion of the Tribe of Judah" that means Jesus Christ.

The key:

> *"No injury whatever was found on him, because he believed in his God.* Daniel 6:23b (NKJV)

The underlying theme of the entire Bible is what God does for those who trust Him. It was not because he was special, one of God's pets, elected or ordained. (See: Heb. 11:4, 5, 7, 8, 22, 32, 33)

Why does God let these things happen? Who's the star of the story? Daniel? Darius? The lions? No, all these are the supporting actors in this great drama.

> *I make a decree that in every dominion of my kingdom men must tremble and fear before the God of Daniel. For He is the living God, And steadfast forever; His kingdom is the one which shall not be destroyed, And His dominion shall endure to the end. He delivers and rescues, And He works signs and wonders In heaven and on earth, Who has delivered Daniel from the power of the lions.* Daniel 6:26-27 (NKJV)

That is a pagan king giving praise to our God. The purpose of this story is to glorify God. Your "lion's den" experience is always that God might be glorified through it.

Success after 90!

> *So this Daniel prospered in the reign of Darius and in the reign of Cyrus the Persian.* Daniel 6:28 (NKJV)

> *But He knows the way that I take; When He has tested me, I shall come forth as gold.* Job 23:10 (NKJV)

Blessed is the man who endures temptation for when he has been approved, he will receive the crown of life which the Lord has promised to those who love Him.
James 1:12

God's purpose in trials is to purify us and bless us:

The following is the story of the imprisonment of John Bunyan, Author of "Pilgrim's Progress." He was imprisoned under the reign of Charles II. If Bunyan had been willing to sign a statement, saying he would not preach in public, he could have been released from prison. Amazingly, if at any time during his twelve years of imprisonment, he had said that he would not preach in public, they would have released him on the day that he said it. So every day of his imprisonment, he had a pardon in his hands if only he would refuse to preach. During those twelve years, Bunyan had a dependent wife and little children. One of his daughters, Mary, was blind. Bunyan was heard to say, "Oh, my poor blind one what sorrow thou art likely to have in this life. Oh, little Mary thou must go naked and hungry and beg on the streets, and be beaten and starved. And I cannot so much as think that the winds should blow on thee." But John Bunyan remained in the dungeon. He gave over his concerns—blind daughter and all—to the keeping of God. Toward the end of his imprisonment he wrote that glorious passage, where he said, "If it shall please God to let frail life last that long, the moss shall grow on my eyebrows before I surrender my principles or violate my conscience." Where are the Bunyans? Where are the Daniels? Where are the men and women who realize that life is not important if the only thing important about it is physical well-being and safety? These men realized that obedience to the principles of God was the highest commitment that a man could make in his life. God asks us to live honestly before a watching world and be unashamed to give testimony of our faith in Jesus Christ. Are you willing to do that?

(56)

Devotions

From the daily devotional *My Utmost for His Highest* by Oswald Chambers
The devotional for February 5th I did on June 30, 2007

Yes, and if I am being poured out as a drink offering on the sacrifice and service of your faith, I am glad and rejoice with you all. Philippians 2:17 (NKJV)

The devotion asked, "Are you willing to sacrifice yourself for the work of another believer—to pour out your life sacrificially for the ministry and faith of others?" Or do you say, "I am not willing to be poured out right now, and I do not want God to tell me how to serve Him. I want to choose the place of my own sacrifice. And I want to have certain people watching me and saying, 'Well done.'"

It is one thing to follow God's way of service if you are regarded as a hero, but quite another thing if the road marked out for you by God requires becoming a 'door mat' under other people's feet. God's purpose may be to teach you to say, 'I know how to be abased...Philippians 4:12. Are you ready to be sacrificed like that? Are you ready to be less than a mere drop in the bucket—to be so totally insignificant that no one remembers you even if they think of those you served? Are you willing to give and be poured out until you are used up and exhausted—not seeking to be ministered to, but to minister? Some saints cannot do menial work while maintaining a saintly attitude, because they feel such service is beneath their dignity."

I looked up abased in the *Webster's Encyclopedia Dictionary of the English Language* and this is what it defined abase as: to humble or dishonor; reduce in rank or standing.

My prayer that day was:

Abba, I am ready to be Your "door mat." I do not know how to be abased, but now I am willing to even be abased if that is Your will for my life. I am ready to be sacrificed like that. I am willing to give and be poured out until I am exhausted and used up. Help me not to look at how I can be ministered to, but how can I minister to others. In Jesus Name, Amen.

I know how to be abased, and I know how to abound.
Everywhere and in all things I have learned both to be
full and to be hungry, both to abound and to suffer need.
I can do all things through Christ who strengthens me.
Philippians 4:12-13 (NKJV)

So whether there is plenty, abundance, and you are well fed or you go hungry, you live to glorify God. If you have sufficiency and enough to spare or you have to go without and be in want, you can live at peace with God. I gain strength from Christ who empowers me to go through all things. Therefore, I am ready for anything through Him who infuses inner strength to me to be self-sufficient in Christ's sufficiency.

The next day in the same journal was the following: I did it the same day as the other devotional.

For I am already being poured out as a drink offering…
2 Timothy 4:6A (NKJV)

The journal said:

"Are you ready to be poured out as an offering? It is an act of your will, not your emotions. Tell God you are ready to be offered as a sacrifice for Him. Then accept the consequences as they come, without any complaints, in spite of what God may send your way. God sends you through a crisis in private, where no other person can help you. From the outside your life may appear the same, but the difference is taking place in your will. Once you have experienced the crises in your will, you will take no thought of the cost when it begins to affect you externally. If you do not deal with God on the level of your will first, the result will be only to arouse sympathy for yourself.

Bind the sacrifice with cords to the horns of the altar.
Psalm 118:27B (NKJV)

You must be willing to be placed on the altar and go through the fire; willing to experience what the altar represents—burning, purification, and separation for only one purpose—the elimination of every desire and affection not grounded in or directed toward God. But you do not eliminate it. God does.

You "bind the sacrifice... to the horns of the altar" and see to it that you do not wallow in self-pity once the fire begins. After you have gone through the fire, there will be nothing that will be able to trouble or depress you. When another crisis arises, you will realize that things cannot touch you as they used to do. What fire lies ahead in your life?

Are you ready to be poured out as an offering to God? Tell God you are ready to be poured out as an offering and God will prove Himself to be all you ever dreamed He would be."

Abba, Father, my DADDY, You are everything and more, so much more than I ever knew You could be to me. I praise You, You have filled full my dreams and longings. I find You to be the center of Your universe. You calm my fears and dry my tears. You strengthen my weaknesses. I find You extremely true to every promise You ever made in Your Word, the Bible.

You meet my needs. You love me in areas I did not even know I needed loving. You are more, More, More! You satisfy me and fill me full to overflowing. I love You. I thank You. I praise You, Abba, my DADDY, Jesus my Christ and God the Holy Spirit. I praise Your Holy Trinity. I am ready to be a poured out offering to You. Bind me with Your cords to the horns of Your altar in heaven. Drag me back if I even try to wander away from You. I need You. I ask in Jesus Blessed Name, Amen.

(57)

Updates

This past summer I joined a Dinner for eight group that meets in homes. We had more in our D-4-8 group than just eight people. We met four times during the summer. We divided into groups and had meals together. Either the host family would provide everything or we would all bring something to eat that night. We met new people from our church. We ate together and visited with each other. We got to know each other by spending some time with them.

We met May 13, 2010 at Michael and Stephanie's house. It was called dinner for eight, but we had a much larger group than that because of all the kids.

While I was at D-4-8 one night Stephanie told me they had a car to sell. Michael had bought the car for their son, Lucas. Lucas decided he wanted a pickup truck instead of the car. So they were selling the car. I told them I was interested. So Michael sold the car to me. Michael had been driving it to work, so I knew the car was dependable. I did not worry about buying a "lemon" because he had checked it out.

Because I went to the Crown Financial meetings about three years ago, I changed my spending patterns. I closed all my credit cards except one. I always paid off the balance in full every month. I went to my bank and got a loan and bought the car. I found out from the bank I had a very good credit rating. I bought the '99 model Honda Accord instead of a new car. The bank set me up to pay it off in three years. Michael said the only thing that did not work on the car was the C D player. Well, now even the C D player works on it, praise God. It needs a new paint job, but I can wait until I can afford that.

Abba, thank You and I praise You for the car. Thank You that Michael and Stephanie sold it to me. Thank You their son did not want it. Thank You that it gets good gas mileage, so I do not have to fill it up often. Thank You that after Bro. Randy needed his car back You supplied the need, and You got me a car of my own. Help me pay for it early. In Jesus Name, Amen.

*****

This month we signed up to do D-4-8 again. They will divide us up into new groups. We had about thirty sign up the first time and this time there are about fifty. It is a great way to get to know the people you just see at church.

*****

I am driving in Wichita now. I am gradually learning my way around town. Momma had an operation on her arm and she cannot drive, so I am driving for her and she tells me which way to go. Each week we go to town to get groceries for the Wednesday night fellowship suppers.

*****

On Dec. 16th I went to Jen and Jeff's for Christmas and came back on the 28th of Dec. Jen and Jeff paid for me to fly to St. Louis. Uncle Kyle, Daddy and Momma took me to the DFW Airport. After I landed I could not find Jen. I called her on my cell phone. Back and forth we called each other. Finally Jen told me to step out into the garage and tell her what level I was on. I told her yellow level and it was only a few more minutes till she drove up to pick me up. I praise God for cell phones.

I had a wonderful time. I watched the girls learn to ice skate at the Olympic Center. Jen and I went shopping before Christmas. It snowed a few days before Christmas. We had a lovely time at Megan's house for Christmas Eve. Christmas morning was special as we opened all of our gifts. Jen cooked a wonderful meal that evening. After Christmas we went shopping with Jen, Jeff, Mackenzie, and Lena as we tried to catch all the after Christmas sales. We tried to work a puzzle and played Phase Ten card games.

I was supposed to drive back halfway with Jen and meet Nanny at Joplin so she could see the kids. But Jen and Nanny talked and decided to fly me back to OK City where Nanny would pick me up. It was a good flight. But I could not find Nanny when I landed. I took two of my three bags off of the baggage turnstile. I could not handle all three of my bags, so I left my big one there. I called Nanny several times. I finally prayed to find Nanny. She called Jen and Jen told her to walk inside the door. I stopped to ask a lady for help. She said I would have to wait a few minutes. I looked down and there was my big bag I had left and the lady was about to put it in baggage claim. So I got my other bag and looked up and there was Nanny standing at the door not very far away. I praise God for answered prayer.

*****

In January of 2012 I had breast cancer. I opted for a mastectomy. I did not have to have chemo or radiation. I have done well. I thank and praise my God I am well. Dr. Myers is my doctor and all the people on staff there treated me with love and compassion.

*****

I have had good results with the new medicine I started taking. It is trial and error to find the right medicines for your body. What works for me may not work for you. It is important to give the medicine enough time for your body to adjust. Allow time for the side effects to lessen or go away and time for you and your doctor to talk about how the medicine is affecting you. Do not give up if at first you do not get the desired outcome. It may take months for medications to help. It may take more than one medicine. Your doctor needs to see and hear from you how you are doing on it.

Abba, thank You and I praise You. Thank You that I am doing so much better now. Thank You for how You got words to paper. It helped me to write this. Thank You for the book. Thank You that You would not let me go to another. Thank You that You are always there to talk to no matter what time of the day or night. Thank You for Your Word. Thank You for the car. Thank You for those who will read this book. Heal them too. Please save people who read this book. I love You and I praise You. In Jesus Name, Amen.

*****

Billie, Cindy, and Jacquetta have read the book and have helped so much to get it into a readable form. Carolyn and Dr. Snowden have read the book. Kathleen, our new secretary at church, and Heather our Finance secretary, have helped me so much to get it into printed form. Thank you to all of them.

Thank you for listening. You have been a part of the healing in me that has taken place as a result of writing this. It is not behind closed doors anymore. I hope and pray it has been a time of healing for you too. Most of all I pray you see God differently than when you started reading this book and that you have come into a time of salvation and now you trust Jesus Christ with your life and future. He is the only way to be saved, all else fails and falls short of the glory of God.

Jesus said to him, "I am the way, the truth, and the life. No one comes to the Father except through Me. John 14:6 (NKJV)

Jesus is the only way to Heaven. Jesus is the only truth that really matters. Jesus is abundant life that lasts forever. Praise God!

CPSIA information can be obtained at www.ICGtesting.com
Printed in the USA
LVOW061232191112

307982LV00002B/4/P